Dear Miriam
Don't be afraid
to get out of live

Are Your Hormones Making You Sick?

A Woman's Guide to Better Health Through Hormonal Balance

Eldred B. Taylor, M.D.
Ava Bell-Taylor, M.D.

Author's Note: This book is not intended to replace a one-on-one relationship with a qualified health care professional and is not intended as medical advice, but as a sharing of knowledge and information from research and experience of the authors. You are advised and encouraged to consult with your healthcare professional with regard to matters relating to your health, and in particular regarding symptoms that may require diagnosis or immediate attention.

Author's note: Unless it is explicitly otherwise stated, the personal details of the experiences shared by women in this book have all been changed to protect their identities, but the essential experiences remain the same.

Visit our Web site at www.physiciansnatmed.com

Printed in the United States of America

First Printing: October 2000
Published by Physicians Natural Medicine Inc.
Second Printing: April 2002
Published by Physicians Natural Medicine Inc.
Third Printing: August 2003
Published by Physicians Natural Medicine Inc.
Distributed by: Biblio Distribution
www.bibliodistribution.com

<u>Dedication</u>

This book is dedicated to

"The Sister's Network"

A group of courageous breast cancer survivors, who have greatly enriched our lives.

Acknowledgements

In Loving Memory of:

Rev. Moses Taylor
Alonzo and Clarice Wyatt
Beatrice Simmons
Ann Stein
Dr. Lacy Bell

Special thanks to the inspiration provided by:

Dr. and Mrs. Walter Kimbrough
Dr. John Daniel Thompson
Dr. John Maxwell
Joyce Meyer

With Great Appreciation to:

Our Creator, without whom this book
could have never been possible

CONTENTS

Introduction

I first became aware of the importance of estrogen and progesterone balance after the birth of my second child. Now in my late thirties, I recently began experiencing severe PMS symptoms. Prior to this time, I had typical PMS symptoms two weeks prior to my period, which included bloating, cravings, leg pain, breast tenderness and pain, irritability, mood swings, insomnia, and headaches. Motrin® relieved most of my symptoms, and I occasionally took Benedryl® to help me sleep at night. My symptoms were tolerable and didn't interfere with my life significantly. However, my symptoms gradually became worse. I began having migraine headaches for two to three days each month. My insomnia worsened and I eventually needed Xanax® at night to sleep. I used St. John's Wort, Valerian Root, and Kava Kava to treat my depression and anxiety. I was on two anti-hypertensive medications to control my blood pressure. I was tired all the time and frequently experienced crying spells for no apparent reason. As you can imagine, this was very distressing for me, a psychiatrist, whose occupation is to help patients suffering from depression and anxiety. I was depressed and in need of some answers. Initially, I thought my symptoms were due to the stress of being in private practice and having two small children, who demanded much of my time. I cut back on my working hours, hoping that it would alleviate my stress. My stress decreased, but my symptoms did not. My husband, an Ob-Gyn, tried to be supportive. He always knew when my periods were about to come and tried to keep the kids from bothering me. I eventually grew sick of myself. I was impatient with my kids, whom I love dearly. I often times apologized to my children for my short temper. I was afraid that my children were beginning to think that there was something wrong with them. I tried to avoid my family on really bad days and forced myself to go into the office. I began exercising three times a week, which seemed to help my symptoms. I also began to feel better as I lost weight. One day as my husband and I were driving along, I noticed a tape lying on the dashboard. I inquired about the content of the tape. He informed me that a patient had given it to him, but he had not had time to listen to it. The tape interested me because it was about the use of natural progesterone to treat hormonal imbalances. My husband's patient shared with him that a natural progesterone cream had helped alleviate most of her PMS symptoms. My husband didn't know much about natural progesterone at that time. I decided to listen to the tape as we drove. While listening to that tape, I realized that perhaps I was progesterone-deficient or may have been experiencing symptoms of estrogen excess. I asked my husband how I could obtain a progesterone cream. Hopeful that it might help me, he agreed to do further research. My husband was surprised to find numerous medical articles written about progesterone creams. Laboratory testing using saliva revealed that my estrogen level was elevated and my progesterone level was decreased. After determining that it was a safe and scientifically sound treatment, my husband started me on a progesterone cream. We also changed our diet to reduce our estrogen exposure. My family and I began eating a diet rich in vegetables, fruits, whole grain breads and pasta, free-range poultry, and fish. We no longer consumed dairy products, but instead used soy substitutes. We all felt better. My daughter, who had suffered from recurrent conjunctivitis and sinusitis, was now well. My son no longer experienced bouts of asthma. I was able to discontinue the two anti-hypertension medications, which I needed to control my blood pressure. My symptoms gradually disappeared and I became my old self again. My energy returned. I was able to sleep at night, and my anxiety and depression diminished. The bloating, leg pain, and headaches were now gone.

My story is the story of thousands of American women who suffer from symptoms of estrogen excess and/or progesterone deficiency. This book was written to enlighten women who are ˙ suffering needlessly. It is our hope that by reading this book, you will gain a better understanding of how diet and lifestyle choices affect your hormonal status.

Hormonal imbalances have created numerous illnesses for women, including PMS, fibroids, endometriosis, fibrocystic breast disease, breast cancer, heart disease, perimenopause, and menopause. By making the right choices, you can restore your body to the balance and good health that God intended you to have.

Ava Bell-Taylor, MD

Chapter 1

Achieving Balance Through

The Menstrual Cycle

All of nature is governed by cycles. The rising and setting of the sun and the changing of seasons occur in cycles. Cycles create balance. When cycles occur out of balance, it can result in extreme weather, pestilence, overpopulation, and illness. Nature desires balance and achieves it through predictable cycles. The menstrual cycle is very important in creating a balance in women. To appreciate the significance of estrogen and progesterone balance, it is important to first understand the menstrual cycle.

The presence and absence of the menstrual cycle defines the reproductive and non-reproductive years of women, respectively. We will discuss the normal sequence of the menstrual cycle to help you understand the significance of two hormones, estrogen and progesterone. Later, we will discuss the illnesses that result when the menstrual cycle is out of balance.

The menstrual cycle's function is to prepare for and maintain a fetus. There are four phases of the menstrual cycle.

Four Phases of the Menstrual Cycle

1. **Menstruation (shedding)**

2. **Follicular or Proliferative Phase (growth)**

3. **Ovulation (release of egg)**

4. **Luteal Phase (development)**

The menstrual cycle starts with menstruation. The first day of bleeding is day one of the menstrual cycle. Menstruation results when a pregnancy does not occur during the previous cycle. Estrogen and progesterone are low during this time and the uterus sheds its tissue.

Following menses (blood flow), the uterus begins to prepare for a possible pregnancy. The pituitary gland, a gland in the brain, begins this preparation by sending a message to the ovary. An egg develops under the influence of follicular stimulating hormone (FSH), produced by the pituitary gland, and estrogen made by the ovary. Estrogen is also responsible for the re-growth of the uterine tissue shed during the previous menses. The development of the egg and the re-growth of the uterine lining are the two primary events of the first 14 days of the menstrual cycle. This part of the cycle is referred to as the follicular stage because of the development of the follicle or the proliferative stage because the uterine lining proliferates, or grows, during this stage.

The next event is ovulation. Ovulation occurs when an egg is released from the ovary and then travels down the fallopian tube for possible fertilization. The egg is released from a cyst, called a follicular cyst that forms in the ovary. Follicular cysts are normal in women during reproductive years. Ovulation is complex and requires the cooperation of hormonal signals from the brain and ovary in order to be carried out successfully. Ovulation can be disrupted by mental or physical stress. Stress can disrupt any or all of the mechanisms involved in ovulation.

After ovulation occurs, the cyst, which housed the egg prior to ovulation, is transformed into the corpus luteum. The corpus luteum is responsible for producing progesterone. Progesterone has many functions. Progesterone maintains and stabilizes the uterine lining during pregnancy. Progesterone instructs the uterine lining to stop growing and start developing and maturing. This maturation must take place to sustain a pregnancy. The corpus luteum is the timekeeper for menstruation and normally functions for 14 days. For 14 days, progesterone is produced while waiting for a fertilized egg. If a woman becomes pregnant, the corpus luteum remains active and produces progesterone until approximately the tenth week of pregnancy. Afterwards, the placenta is able to make its own progesterone.

If pregnancy does not occur, the corpus luteum degenerates. Progesterone production decreases drastically. The uterine lining, which is no longer supported by progesterone, detaches and begins to shed, thus starting menses again.

Each month a woman's body goes through the following cycle:
1. Menses - bleeding and shedding of the uterine lining. **Estrogen and progesterone levels are low.**
2. Growth – re-growth of lining of uterus, growth of a new egg, and breast growth. **Estrogen is the dominant hormone.**
3. Release of an egg for fertilization - **Estrogen and progesterone are working in partnership.**
4. Development and maturation of uterine lining and breasts in preparation for pregnancy - **Progesterone is dominant.**

This is a simplified overview of the menstrual cycle. Estrogen and progesterone are the principal hormones involved in the menstrual cycle but their effects encompass much more than the regulation of the menstrual cycle. To appreciate the importance of estrogen and progesterone balance, we must first review the functions of these two diverse hormones.

Points to Remember

- Estrogen is made during the first half of the menstrual cycle.
- Progesterone is made during the second half of the menstrual cycle.
- Progesterone cannot be produced without ovulation.
- Estrogen and progesterone must work in partnership if a normal menstrual cycle is to occur.

Chapter 2

Hormones 101: A Beginner's Course

Hormones function as messengers in the body. Hormones are released from glands and travel by way of the bloodstream to specific organs that are able to respond to their messages. A cell cannot respond to a hormone's message unless it contains a receptor for that hormone. Hormones and receptors fit together like a lock and key. Certain cells have locks that only a specific hormone can unlock. Receptors are very sensitive. The receptor will only respond completely to its designated hormone. If the hormone has a slight change in structure, the receptor will detect the change. The receptor may respond partially to the modified hormone, but its normal response will be altered, usually resulting in negative side effects.

Hormones and receptors are present in plants, animals and humans. Some hormones have very similar structures, even though they are found in different species. Naturally occurring hormones can cross react with different species. For example, phytoestrogens, or plant estrogens, can stimulate human estrogen receptors.

Steroid hormones must penetrate the membranes surrounding the cell in order to attach to the receptor inside the cell. The cell membrane is made out of fat-like substances called fatty acids. To pass through the cell membrane, the hormone must be able to penetrate the fatty acids comprising the membrane. Steroid hormones, or sex hormones, are made from cholesterol, which allows them to penetrate cell membranes. Once through the membrane, the hormone is able to attach to the receptor and deliver its message. Approximately 99% of steroid hormones are bound to water-soluble proteins, which allows them to be transported in the blood. These carrier proteins inactivate the hormone but allow it to be transported easily in the bloodstream, which is mostly water. The approximate 1% of the hormone that is not attached to a carrier protein is able to travel inside the cell to deliver its message. Later in this book, we will discuss factors that determine how much free hormone is available to female target tissues.

Estrogen

No hormone has been studied as much as estrogen. During the 1950's, a physician wrote the book *Forever Young*. This book suggested that the lack of estrogen was responsible for premature aging in women. Since that time, an incredible amount of research, money, and advertising has been directed towards supporting this assumption. However, recent evidence now points to the fact that most women in the U.S. are either experiencing symptoms of estrogen excess or of progesterone deficiency.

Estrogen is a sex steroid hormone. It is transported in the blood by a carrier protein to the appropriate tissue sites. When estrogen finds a cell with the appropriate receptor it attaches itself to that cell and delivers its message.

Estrogen's message to the target tissue cells is GROW and MULTIPLY. This message is conveyed intensely to the uterus, ovaries and the breasts. The message to the inner lining of the uterus is to grow, multiply, and replace the layer of tissue that was shed during the previous menses. A similar message is communicated to the breasts. The breast cells are stimulated to grow, multiply, and prepare for a possible pregnancy. Estrogen stimulates the ovaries to make follicles, which produce eggs. Estrogen also stimulates the vaginal tissue and the lower part of the bladder. It keeps these tissues strong, moist, and well functioning and promotes normal vaginal lubrication. Without estrogen, the vagina becomes dry, sensitive, and more prone to infection and bladder function declines.

During puberty, estrogen is responsible for the development of secondary sex characteristics. The increase in estrogen production during puberty causes pubic hair to grow, breasts to bud and grow, and the uterus to completely develop in preparation for menstruation.

Estrogen also conveys messages to other parts of the body. The bone has receptors for estrogen. Bone cells, called osteoclasts, contain estrogen receptors. Osteoclasts are responsible for breaking down old bone. Bone is constantly being destroyed and replaced. Estrogen slows down the destruction of old bone by inhibiting osteoclasts. We will discuss estrogen's effect on bone in more detail when we discuss osteoporosis.

Estrogen can also influence other hormones. Sex steroid hormone receptors are very similar in structure to thyroid hormone receptors. Thyroid hormone is responsible for regulating metabolism, weight and energy levels. Estrogen can increase thyroid binding globulin (thyroid carrier protein) and block the effect of thyroid hormone. This estrogen effect is important during the menstrual cycle because it decreases metabolism, allowing the body to store fat that can be used for energy during the pregnancy. Estrogen increases the secretion of aldosterone. Aldosterone increases salt and water retention, which protects the body against dehydration. Estrogen increases the pituitary gland's secretion of prolactin, which stimulates breast cell growth and milk production.

Estrogen also effects mood and cognition, or the ability to think clearly. Clinical practice and studies done in rats show that too little or too much estrogen can cause changes in mood and cognition. Women who are menopausal and have decreased estrogen levels will experience mood swings and poor concentration. This is also true of women with elevated estrogen levels. Estrogen must be present in an optimal concentration and in proper relationship to progesterone for women to function at their best.

Functions of Estrogen

- Regrowth of uterine lining
- Maintains vaginal and bladder tissue health
- Stimulates growth of breast cells
- Is responsible for female sex organ development during puberty
- Decreases bone breakdown
- Effects mood, cognition, and concentration
- Decreases thyroid function, which slows metabolism and increases fat storage

All Estrogen is Not Created Equally

Estrogen is usually referred to in books, in magazines, and by healthcare professionals, as a single substance. However, there are several forms of estrogen that can attach to the estrogen receptors. The main difference between the estrogen types is the amount of time it stays bound to the receptor. The longer the binding time is, the more potent the estrogen. Weak estrogens provide a low, safe stimulation of the cell, while strong estrogens have an effect similar to attaching a car battery to a 9-volt transistor radio. We will discuss some of the most common estrogens found inside and outside the body and their effects on the body. We will start by discussing the weakest estrogen and progress to the strongest.

Phytoestrogens are plant estrogens. The most intensely studied phytoestrogen is soy. It was mentioned earlier that plants and animals produce hormones that behave like human hormones. These hormones can bind to hormone receptors in human cells producing a biological response. Phytoestrogens are weak estrogens. They bind to the estrogen receptor for a short period of time, and provide minimal stimulation to the estrogen receptor located in the cells. They can provide adequate stimulation to estrogen-sensitive cells in estrogen-deficient women. Phytoestrogens can also provide protection against stronger or excessive amounts of estrogen. Phytoestrogens, when consumed in appropriate amounts can fill the estrogen receptor, resulting in the blockage of stronger estrogens that may attach and communicate a harmful message.

Estriol is the weakest estrogen produced by women. Estriol is at its highest concentration during pregnancy. Estriol in a non-pregnant woman is made as a by-product of estradiol, which is a much stronger estrogen. Estriol had been ignored and considered unimportant until recently. Studies are now showing that estriol in appropriate concentrations can provide all the benefits of estrogen replacement without increasing the risk of breast cancer. Some studies show that estriol and phytoestrogens actually protect the breast from cancer by blocking estrogen receptors. By making estrogen receptors unavailable to stronger estrogen, phytoestrogens and estriol may prevent stronger estrogens from stimulating potential cancer cells.

Estrone is a moderately strong estrogen produced by the body. It is primarily made from androstenedione, a steroid hormone made in the adrenal gland. Androstenedione is a male hormone (androgen). However, in women it is metabolized into the two female sex hormones, estrone and estradiol. Androgens are converted into estrone and estradiol in fat, skin, muscle tissue, and the uterus. It is believed that elevated levels of estrone in obese women may increase their risk of breast cancer.

Estradiol, which is made in the ovaries, is the strongest estrogen found in the body. Estradiol stimulates the estrogen receptor more than estriol or estrone because it attaches more tightly to the receptor, and it remains bound for a longer period of time. Estradiol is primarily responsible for replenishing the uterine lining after each menses. A surge of estradiol is also needed to stimulate ovulation. Synthetic estradiol is primarily used in hormone replacement and birth control pills.

Premarin® is a widely prescribed drug, which contains conjugated estrogens. Its origin is described in its name. Premarin® is derived from pregnant mare urine. The types of estrogens found in Premarin® have not been completely identified. In the medical literature, it is described as conjugated equine estrogen. Premarin®

is a widely prescribed drug because it has been studied, advertised, and made commercially available longer than other forms of hormonal replacement.

Xenoestrogens are the most potent estrogens. Taken from the word *xeno*, meaning "new in existence or manmade," these estrogens are not found in the human body or anywhere else in the plant or animal kingdom, but are by-products of commercial compounds. Many pesticides and organic solvents, which are found in cleaners and pollutants, behave like estrogen when consumed or absorbed by the human body. In isolation, these chemicals are usually found in small quantities that are not harmful. However, when small quantities of multiple xenoestrogens are combined, they have a synergistic effect. They amplify the effect of each other. Combined xenoestrogens can have an effect that is 100 to 1000 times more potent than estradiol, the strongest estrogen made in the body. Many of the pesticides like DDT have been banned because of their harmful effects. Unfortunately, DDT can remain active in the soil for more than 25 years. This allows DDT to remain present in the food supply long after its use has been banned. Despite the United States DDT ban, we import produce from countries that have not banned this pesticide.

What Influences Estrogen Activity?

- **Estrogen Binding to SHBG (carrier protein)**

- **Estrogen Production**

- **Estrogen Metabolism & Elimination**

- **External Estrogen Exposure**

Sex Hormone Binding Globulin (SHBG) is the protein that carries the majority of estrogen in the bloodstream. Estrogen, which is fat soluble, must be attached to SHBG, a water-soluble protein, while it is being transported to target tissues. Another water-soluble protein, called albumin, binds 10% to 40% of estrogen. Only 1% of estrogen is unbound or free. The free estrogen is able to deliver its message to the cells that contain estrogen receptors.

SHBG controls the amount of active hormone available to target tissues. Therefore, it is important to know what factors control SHBG levels. Hyperthyroidism, pregnancy and estrogen increase SHBG levels. Weight, insulin, low fat, high fiber diets, cortisol, progestins, and growth hormone decrease SGBG. Factors that decrease SHBG increase the amount of free estrogen available. Conversely, factors that increase SHBG decrease the amount of free estrogen available.

Estrogen is produced from cholesterol via a multi-step process. Cholesterol, ovulation, and body fat each play an integral role in the production of estrogen. Fat tissue is a predominant source of estrogen production. As your body weight increases, so does your estrogen production. Conversely, as your weight declines, so does your estrogen production. Women, who are no longer ovulating, such as menopausal women or those who have had their ovaries surgically removed, may experience a decline in estrogen production if adequate fat tissue is not present. Diets that severely restrict fat and cholesterol intake may also diminish estrogen production.

The metabolism and elimination of estrogen influences the total amount of estrogen available in the body. After estradiol attaches to a receptor and delivers its message, it is released back into the bloodstream and may attach to other cell receptors before being eliminated. If estradiol does not reattach, it is metabolized to estriol, a less active compound. The primary site of estrogen metabolism is the liver. The liver requires certain vitamins and minerals to properly deactivate estradiol. The B vitamins, Vitamin E, magnesium, and substances like indole 3-carbinol, found in vegetables such as broccoli and cauliflower, are needed for estrogen metabolism. Deficiencies in these vitamins and minerals can affect estrogen metabolism and increase free estrogen levels. Even after the metabolized estrogen is transported to the large bowel for elimination the final step in deactivation cannot be performed if the normal bowel bacteria are not present. The partially metabolized estrogen can then be reabsorbed back into the bloodstream. Normal bowel bacteria can be destroyed by overuse of antibiotics and diets that lack the proper amount of whole, unprocessed foods. As you can see, even small amounts of estrogen can have an extended and cumulative effect on the body.

Finally, external estrogen exposure can influence estrogen activity. Estrogen influences its own receptors. The more estrogen present in the body, the more estrogen receptors the body makes. This is somewhat unusual for a steroid hormone. Most steroid hormones decrease the number of receptors in the body when levels are elevated. However, in the case of estrogen, the body increases its ability to respond to estrogen by making more receptors. The body has an unlimited ability to respond to estrogen. This unique phenomenon may play a role in the development of cancer in women, particularly when progesterone is low or absent.

Excess Estrogen

Excess estrogen can cause or make worse:
- Irregular/heavy bleeding
- Breast tenderness
- Depression, fatigue, and poor concentration
- Fibrocystic breast
- PMS
- Decreased libido
- Fibroid growth
- Endometriosis
- Water retention and bloating
- Fat gain around hips and thighs
- Breast and uterine cancer

Estrogen Deficiency

Decreased estrogen can cause or make worse:
- Vaginal dryness
- Decreased sex drive
- Disturbed sleep
- Poor concentration
- Depression
- Thinning skin

Progesterone

Progesterone is a steroid hormone. It has 21 carbon atoms while estrogen has only 19. It is a precursor, or building block, for estrogen but also conveys its own unique message to cells. Estrogen directs cells to grow and multiply, while progesterone directs them to slow their growth and mature normally. Progesterone controls and modifies the message of estrogen.

Progesterone is produced only by the corpus luteum; the cyst that remains after the egg is expelled during ovulation. Unlike estrogen, progesterone is not made by the conversion of other steroid hormones in peripheral tissue, such as fat, skin and muscle. Progesterone production occurs only after ovulation.

Progestins are synthetic versions of progesterone. Progestins have a chemical make-up similar to progesterone. These compounds bind to the progesterone receptors in cells but they are unable to deliver the entire message. They are only able to direct the cell to perform a limited amount of the progesterone message. The hormone receptor complex is very specific. If one carbon atom of progesterone is changed, the message to the target tissue is also changed. Progesterone is metabolized to estrogen, testosterone and cortisol in women. Progestins, altered progesterone molecules, can create a roadblock in this cascade. The altered structure of progestins not only affects the progesterone message; it also results in unwanted side effects. However, the short-term use of Progestins is helpful in treating vaginal bleeding and protecting the uterus from cancer caused by estrogen exposure.

Functions of Progesterone

- **Promote and maintain pregnancy**
- **Diuretic; decreases water retention**
- **Increases thyroid function**
- **Natural antidepressant and anti-anxiety hormone**
- **Increases libido**
- **Decreases uterine contractions (cramping)**
- **Decreases estrogen receptors**
- **Promotes cell maturation**
- **Decreases cell multiplication caused by estrogen**
- **Promotes normal cell death**
- **Decrease frequency of seizures**

The word progesterone is derived from two words, promote and gestation. Progesterone is the only hormone needed to maintain a pregnancy. Progesterone is made after ovulation. Its function is to develop and mature the lining of the uterus so that it can sustain a pregnancy. Progesterone made by the corpus luteum sustains the pregnancy until the placenta is able to make enough progesterone to maintain the pregnancy. The placenta makes an enormous amount of progesterone. The body normally makes 2 to 4 milligrams a day of progesterone, but during pregnancy the body makes 200 to 400 milligrams a day of progesterone.

Many infertility specialists use progesterone suppositories when treating women with infertility problems. Women who are deficient in progesterone may have frequent early miscarriages. The addition of progesterone will often allow the uterus to maintain the early pregnancy until the placenta takes over the production of progesterone. Progesterone is also used in assisted reproduction or in vitro fertilization. It helps provide an optimal uterine environment in which fertilized eggs can grow. Progestins (synthetically altered progesterone) are not used to maintain pregnancies. The addition of progestins will not maintain a pregnancy and is also associated with cardiac defects in the fetus.

Another major function of progesterone is to regulate the activity of estrogen. We discussed earlier that estrogen increases the production of its own receptors. However, progesterone is able to decrease the production of estrogen receptors. This decreases the cell's ability to overreact to excessive levels of estrogen. This is one of the mechanisms by which progesterone protects the body from estrogen-induced cancers of the uterus and breasts. Another mechanism by which progesterone regulates estrogen is by promoting cell differentiation. Progesterone promotes normal cell development and can override estrogen's message to multiply. Estrogen and progesterone work together better in balance than they do alone or out of balance.

Progesterone blocks the action of a hormone called aldosterone. Aldosterone causes the body to store water in the presence of dehydration. Progesterone blocks aldosterone receptors and allows the body to release excess water. Progesterone behaves like a natural diuretic.

Progesterone decreases thyroid binding globulin. As mentioned earlier, estrogen increases thyroid binding globulin levels, which inactivates thyroid hormone. This slows the body's metabolism and allows the storage of fat and energy for a future fetus. Progesterone, on the other hand, decreases thyroid binding globulin levels, thereby increasing the amount of active thyroid hormone. Thyroid hormone can now stimulate the utilization of the fat stored for energy.

Progesterone is very important to the normal functioning of the brain. A blood brain barrier protects the brain from outside substances. Only what is necessary is allowed to cross this barrier. Over 60% of the progesterone made by the body is concentrated in the brain. In the brain, progesterone can bind to GABA receptors. These receptors are responsible for maintaining an appropriate mood. GABA receptors are the receptors to which antidepressant drugs and anti-anxiety drugs bind to produce their effects. New studies show that these mood-altering drugs work because they elevate the concentration of a progesterone by-product.

Progesterone acts like a natural antidepressant and anti-anxiety drug.

Progesterone also assists in the myelinization of nerve cells. Myelin forms the insulation around nerve cells. Nerves and electrical wires are both alike in that they conduct electrical current. Electrical wires need rubber insulation; nerves need myelin insulation. Insulation allows current to be transmitted without interruption. Seizures are the result of an abnormal flow of electrical current in the brain. Progesterone lowers seizure activity. It decreases the rate of seizures by preventing short circuits, which cause seizures. In general, progesterone seems to increase concentration and allow clearer thinking when present in the proper amount.

Progesterone increases libido, both directly and indirectly. Normally there is a small rise in progesterone prior to ovulation. Studies have shown that woman initiate sex more often immediately prior to ovulation. This may be due to a direct effect of progesterone or an increase in the metabolism of progesterone to testosterone. In either case, progesterone positively affects sex drive.

Progesterone relaxes smooth muscle, which is found in the uterus. Progesterone can relax smooth muscle contraction. The contractions of the uterine smooth muscle during the menstrual cycle are experienced as menstrual cramps. Progesterone can decrease the intensity of menstrual cramps. Smooth muscle also lines blood vessel walls; therefore, progesterone can relax blood vessels. This effect may protect the heart from heart attacks. A study showed that in primates (apes), the addition of progesterone made it relatively impossible to induce heart attacks in these animals. Further study is needed to see if progesterone has the same effect on the human heart.

Progesterone effects bone metabolism. It stimulates a cell in the bone called the osteoblast, which is responsible for new bone formation. The osteoblast uses calcium to form new bone. Bone is constantly in a state of development. Osteoclasts break down old bone, while new bone replaces the old bone under the direction of osteoblasts, which are influenced by progesterone. Estrogen regulates osteoclasts to make sure they do not break down the bone too rapidly.   This is another example of how estrogen and progesterone work together. When progesterone and estrogen are available in their proper relationship, they promote good bone health.

In the absence of sufficient quantities of progesterone, the body begins to make androgens (male hormones) to regulate the effect of estrogen. Androgen production in women produces male pattern baldness and hirsuitism (facial hair). Male pattern baldness includes receding hairlines, bald spots in the back of the head, and thinning hair. This occurs when the ovary is primarily producing testosterone in addition to androgens produced by the adrenal gland.

When ovulation does not occur, progesterone is not produced. Androgens are the only defense against overexposure to estrogen in the absence of progesterone. To understand progesterone's role in hair growth, you need only to examine the hair and nails of a pregnant woman. Most women report that their hair and nails became longer and thicker when pregnant. During pregnancy, the progesterone level is maintained at a maximum level. Unfortunately, women report a reversal of these benefits after delivery.

Progesterone Deficiency

Progesterone deficiency can cause or make worse:
- **Irregular/heavy bleeding**
- **Breast tenderness**
- **Depression, fatigue, and poor concentration**
- **Fibrocystic breast**
- **PMS**
- **Decreased libido**
- **Fibroid growth**
- **Endometriosis**
- **Water retention and bloating**
- **Fat gain around hips and thighs**
- **Bone loss**
- **Hair loss**
- **Breast and uterine cancer**

Progesterone Excess

- **Euphoria**
- **Prolonged excessive use may lead to symptoms of progesterone deficiency**

We have reviewed the function of the menstrual cycle and its two primary hormones, estrogen and progesterone. Hopefully, it is now evident that estrogen and progesterone are needed in balanced amounts to promote optimal health benefits. Later in the book, we will discuss how you can assist your body in maintaining this delicate balance of hormones to avoid potential health problems.

Points to Remember

1. **Balance in the menstrual cycle is essential.**

2. **Estrogen's message to cells is to GROW.**

3. **Progesterone's message to cells is to stop growing and DEVELOP.**

4. **Hormones have checks and balances. Each hormone in the body has a counterpart hormone that regulates its function.**

5. **Estrogen excess and progesterone deficiency can cause identical symptoms in women.**

Chapter 3

Are Your Hormones in Balance?

The Estrogen/Progesterone Ratio

We would like to introduce to you a new way of thinking about estrogen and progesterone. Conventional medicine, pharmaceutical companies, and patients like to categorize solutions in absolute terms. Society likes to classify things as good or bad, healthy or dangerous. Fad diets like to claim that proteins, carbohydrates, fats, fiber, etc., are either good or bad for you. Actually, you need all of these foods in the proper proportion to maintain weight and health. The same is true about hormonal balance. Estrogen is neither bad nor good. The same is true of progesterone, testosterone, DHEA, thyroid hormone, and cortisol. These hormones must be maintained in the proper concentration and ratio to one another. When one is either excessive or deficient, the normal ratio is disturbed and the optimal function of the hormone is altered. This disturbance in the hormonal balance can affect many body systems.

Estrogen and progesterone work best together in their proper ratio. One cannot optimally function without the influence of the other. The normal ratio of free estrogen to free progesterone is approximately 20 to 1 after ovulation, during which time progesterone is the dominant hormone. **Fig. 1**

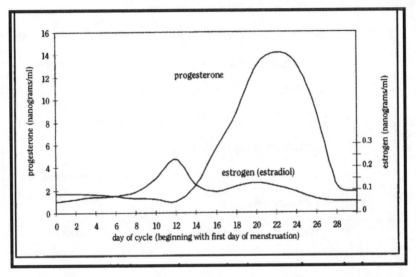

Fig. 1

Progesterone should be 20 times higher than estrogen during the second half of the menstrual cycle. If progesterone is lower or higher than normal, it produces the same clinical symptoms. An excess of estrogen and/or a deficiency of progesterone are responsible for many of the illnesses that afflict women. Hopefully, the information provided in this book will change your way of thinking, or at least challenge you to question the assumption that all women are essentially estrogen-deficient. This chapter will review the factors that play a role in creating these hormonal imbalances.

> ## Women in the U.S
>
> - **80% of women complain of PMS**
> - **20-50% of women have fibroids**
> - **80-90% complain of perimenopausal symptoms**
> - **Premenopausal breast cancer (breast cancer prior to age 50) is increasing**
> - **90% of menopausal women complain of menopausal symptoms**
> - **45% of postmenopausal women are effected by osteoporosis**
> - **Infertility is increasing in men and women**

What Disrupts the Balance?

If balance is required for the ultimate biological response of hormones, did God create women to be out of balance, or are elements in the environment disturbing this hormonal balance? The statistics listed above are unique to women residing in the United States. Women in other countries, who do not share our diet and lifestyles, do not experience the same health problems as women in the U.S. Asian women with traditional Asian diets have minimal menopausal symptoms and breast cancer risk. Conditions such as

PMS and fibroids are infrequent in Asia. Hysterectomies are rarely performed. As countries in Asia, particularly Hong Kong and Japan, have adapted a more American diet and lifestyle, their health statistics are beginning to resemble American statistics. Diet, lifestyle, exposure to external estrogens, delayed childbirth and stress all play a major role in creating hormonal imbalances.

Poor Diet

The traditional American diet consists of high fat, high carbohydrate and low fiber foods. Our foods are processed and contain minimal nutritional value. The American diet poses a constant threat to hormonal balance and functioning.

A high-fat diet increases the amount of fat the body stores. The more fat the body stores, the more estrogen the fat cells make. The type of fat or oils that are consumed is important. Fats, omega 3, 6 and 9 fatty acids, are used to produce the membranes around cells. When cell membranes are made of excessive amounts of omega 6 fatty acids, it magnifies the receptor's response to estrogen. This means that if your estrogen level is normal, but your diet contains primarily omega 6 fatty acids, the cell membrane causes the estrogen receptor to respond in an exaggerated manner.

Omega 6 fatty acids are found in:

- **Hydrogenated and partially hydrogenated oils, which are found in almost all preserved foods**
- **Corn oil**
- **Soybean oil**
- **Sesame oil**
- **Mayonnaise**
- **Commercial salad dressing**
- **Margarine**
- **Almost all fast foods are prepared in Omega 6 oils**

A diet that is high in foods containing simple carbohydrates, white sugar, and white bread rapidly raises insulin levels. When insulin levels remain high for an extended period of time, cells become resistant to insulin. This causes a condition called insulin resistance, which usually leads to diabetes. Insulin intensifies the estrogen signal transmitted to cells. Insulin also decreases the amount of sex hormone binding globulin (SHBG). This allows more free estrogen to be available to the body.

Most of the foods that are available at the grocery store have been processed. Processing is usually done to increase shelf life, enhance flavor, and make the color of the food more appealing. Processing the food usually strips away most of its nutritional value. For example, wheat goes through more than 20 processes before it becomes white bread. One of the initial processes is the removal of the wheat germ, because it causes the bread to spoil rapidly. Unfortunately, all of the nutrients are found in the wheat germ. Estrogen is metabolized in the liver, and it requires a lot of vitamins, minerals, and enzymes found in food to be properly metabolized. If the nutrients have been processed out of the food, it provides little benefit to the body. Without the aid of vitamins, minerals, and enzymes found in unprocessed foods, estrogen metabolism is greatly affected. Americans are consuming large quantities of empty calories. These are calories that can be stored as fat but have little nutritional value.

Fruit and vegetables are important in hormonal metabolism. The predominance of corporate-owned, versus family farms, has changed the way produce is grown. During the process of corporate farming, the soil is turned over rapidly and is not replenished of its trace minerals and vitamins, thus producing fruits and vegetables that are devoid of essential vitamins and minerals. The produce is also sprayed with pesticides and fed fertilizers that behave like estrogens. The combination of vitamin and mineral-depleted soil, pesticides, and fertilizers results in fruits and vegetables that hamper hormone metabolism and contribute to estrogen excess.

Fiber is important for two reasons. Fiber increases SHBG, which is important in deactivating excess estrogen. Remember that increased SHBG levels result in decreased free, active estrogen.

Also, fiber helps to remove estrogen from the body by increasing the frequency of bowel movements. We mentioned earlier that estrogen could perform its function several times before it is metabolized and eliminated. Estrogen, which is delivered to the bowel for elimination, can be reabsorbed if it remains in the bowel for an extended period of time. Women with high fiber diets eliminate up to 50% more estrogen in their feces than women with low fiber diets.

Sedentary Lifestyle

Sedentary lifestyle is commonplace in America and has an adverse effect on hormonal balance. More and more women are becoming heads of households and breadwinners. With this change, come all of the headaches of long office hours. There is little time for physical activity at work or home. Most women are exhausted at the end of the workday and must come home to face the additional responsibilities of caring for children and household duties. Exhausted and sleep deprived, exercise is often placed on the back burner.

Decreased physical activity and poor eating habits lead to weight gain. Sex hormone binding globulin (SHBG) decreases as weight increases and more active estrogen becomes available without a similar rise in progesterone. Insulin levels are higher when we consume more calories than we expend. These excess calories are stored as fat. Insulin intensifies the body's response to estrogen.

Increased estrogen levels compound the weight problem by predisposing women to depression, anxiety, insomnia, fatigue, and additional weight gain.

Excess estrogen can inhibit ovulation. Without ovulation, a woman makes essentially no progesterone, which severely disturbs the estrogen/progesterone ratio. A sedentary lifestyle traps a woman in a vicious cycle of weight gain, estrogen excess, decreased progesterone levels, more weight gain, depression, fatigue, and less activity.

Implementing a simple exercise program of walking or biking 15 minutes a day and gradually increasing to 30 minutes a day can reverse the symptoms of excess estrogen. If this doesn't work for you, try using a beginner's exercise video at home. It may be tough initially, but your energy levels and mood will improve after a few short weeks of activity.

External Estrogen

External estrogen exposure is a very important source of estrogen excess. Let's begin by examining our exposure through food. Estrogen is given to cattle to promote weight gain and water retention. This is beneficial to the cattle farmer because the farmers sell cattle by the pound. The estrogen given to cattle remains stored in the animal fat. When we consume the animal fat, we are exposed to active estrogen. The same cows provide us with milk and dairy products, which also expose us to more estrogen. In addition, chickens are fed estrogen and growth hormone to increase breast size and enhance color. Pesticides and fertilizers that behave like estrogen contaminate fruits and vegetables.

Other sources of estrogen exposure include the xenohormones. As mentioned earlier, these are manmade chemical compounds that behave like hormones. DDT and DES (diethylstilbestrol) are two common xenohormones. DES was given to women in the 1950's and 1960's to prevent miscarriage. The adverse effects of DES were not realized until the daughters of these women were found to have uterine malformations, infertility problems, and increased risk of cervical cancer. Other sources of xenoestrogens are solvents and adhesives found in cleaning supplies and alcohol-based nail polishes and removers. Petroleum based pesticides, herbicides and fungicides, car exhausts, emulsifiers found in soaps and cosmetics, nearly all plastics, and industrial wastes (PCBs and dioxin) contain xenoestrogens. The long-term effects of xenoestrogens are now being manifested. The federal government is beginning to study the possible environmental causes of breast and prostate cancer and other diseases.

Delayed Childbearing

Delaying childbirth after age 30 increases a woman's risk for three female cancers, including breast, ovary, and uterine cancers. When God said to be fruitful and multiply, he may have had the protection of women in mind. The menstrual cycle seems to have one purpose - and one purpose only - and that is to facilitate reproduction. All of the hormonal interactions of the menstrual cycle are geared towards optimizing the body's environment for reproduction.

During pregnancy, progesterone is the predominant hormone, and estriol is the weakest estrogen. Studies have shown that not only are these two hormones protective against cancer, but also the benefits they offer continue with time. In other words, women who become pregnant earlier in life and have more pregnancies benefit from these two hormones in that they are less likely to develop cancer.

One explanation for this protective effect is that pregnancy matures the female reproductive system. The breast and the uterus develop completely during pregnancy. It is believed that cancer-causing agents can change an immature cell into a cancer cell more easily than it could a mature slow-growing cell. The longer the female reproductive system consists of immature cells, the more likely cancer-causing environmental factors can alter these cells. Because estrogen instructs estrogen receptor containing cells to grow, the more menstrual cycles a woman experiences, the more likely potential cancer cells are going to be stimulated by estradiol. If a woman has excess estrogen and low progesterone levels, the risk of cancer increases.

Stress

American women are especially familiar with stress. Women have been cast into very different and demanding roles over the last 30 years. Women are now expected to work outside the home, care for children, spouses, and often times, aging parents. In addition, women must manage baby-sitters, housekeepers, participate in school and extracurricular activities, help with homework, and be involved in community and church activities. When we survey these expectations, we can begin to appreciate the stress that women constantly endure.

The body counters the effects of stress through a process called the stress response. The stress response aids the body in handling the everyday stressors of life. It is an instinctive reflex action that is a part of animal adaptation. However, when stress is extreme, unusual, or long lasting, the stress response can create disturbances of hormonal and bodily functions.

The initial response to stress is the *alarm reaction*, or fight-or-flight response. The body secretes adrenaline and other stress-related hormones. This increases blood flow to the brain, heart, lungs and muscles and increases glucose levels in the blood. All of these functions are necessary for fighting or fleeing a dangerous situation.

The next phase is the *resistance reaction.* During this phase, cortisol is released in order to prolong the changes initiated by the alarm reaction. Cortisol stimulates the conversion of protein to energy, so the body has a large supply of energy after glucose supplies have been depleted. Cortisol also increases sodium levels and elevates blood pressure. The resistance reaction provides the changes required for meeting an emotional crisis, performing strenuous tasks, and fighting infection.

A prolonged resistance reaction, however, can lead to exhaustion. *Exhaustion* is the result of a depleted cortisol supply, which leads to a low blood glucose levels and inadequate energy to cells. The cells also lose potassium, which can lead to cell death. The exhaustion stage results in the weakening of the heart, blood vessels, the adrenal gland, and the immune system. Organs, which have been exposed to tremendous stress, eventually become exhausted and unable to respond adequately. Several studies show that the diagnosis of cancer usually follows a stressful event in the patient's life.

Stress may be the number one cause of menstrual irregularities and anovulatory cycles. Whenever a reproductive age woman comes to my office with a recent change in her normal menstrual cycles, I immediately begin to inquire about stressful events in her life. Starting a new job, starting school, a divorce, death in the family, preparing for a wedding, problems with children, etc., are common stressors, which lead to menstrual abnormalities.

How does stress affect a woman's menses? When a woman is faced with a stressful situation, the stress hormone, cortisol, is released. Cortisol decreases SHBG. This increases the amount of free estrogen. Elevated estrogen levels can block ovulation. When ovulation is blocked, progesterone production is absent. This scenario leads to heavy, irregular menses. In addition to dealing with a stressful situation, she is now faced with the dilemma of what to do about her heavy, irregular menstrual cycles. Is it possible that the bleeding is being caused by cancer, fibroids or cyst? Will surgery be necessary? To make matters worse, her husband begins complaining because she is bleeding all of the time. Her stress is intensified, and the bleeding worsens. This is a classic example of how the mind affects the body. Often times, simply making women aware of the role of stress in creating menstrual irregularities will lead to cessation of their bleeding.

Conditions Related to Stress

Angina (chest pain)
Asthma
Autoimmune diseases
Cancer (i.e. breast cancer)
Cardiovascular disease
Common cold
Depression
Diabetes
Headaches
High blood pressure
Immune suppression
Irritable bowel syndrome
Menstrual irregularities
Premenstrual syndrome
Rheumatoid arthritis

Alcohol

Alcohol damages the liver. The liver is the primary site of estrogen metabolism. Most alcoholics have poor eating habits, which leads to vitamin and mineral deficiencies. As a result, the liver does not have the proper nutrients needed to break down estrogen. Liver cells damaged and destroyed by alcohol, lead to further estrogen metabolism problems. Alcoholic men and women usually have signs and symptoms of estrogen excess. For example, alcoholic men have increased breast size due to the presence of excess estrogen. Only two to four drinks per day can cause significant liver damage.

Many factors are capable of altering the estrogen/progesterone ratio. Now you can appreciate why the symptoms of estrogen/progesterone ratio disturbances are so rampant. They have become so commonplace that many women and doctors consider them normal.

<u>Paradigm Shift</u>

Estrogen deficiency is NOT the primary cause of adolescent, premenopausal and menopausal health problems in women!

Points to Remember

1. The presence of estrogen and progesterone in a proper ratio creates balance in the body.
2. There are many factors that can disrupt the estrogen/progesterone ratio.
3. Modifying diet and lifestyle choices can control many of the risk factors for estrogen/progesterone imbalance

Chapter 4

Salivary Testing:

Diagnosing Estrogen/ Progesterone Ratio Disturbances

Steroid sex hormones dissolve in fat, but not in water. The blood consists of blood cells and serum. Serum primarily consists of water and water-soluble substances like sodium, potassium and calcium. When fat-soluble substances like estrogen are absorbed from the stomach and gut, they are then transported to the liver. Once there, they are attached to a carrier protein that is water-soluble and then released into the blood for transport. Fat-soluble hormones like estrogen and progesterone are inactive when they are connected to the carrier protein. . Sex hormone binding globulin (SHBG), which transports estrogen in the blood, is a major carrier protein for estrogen. The hormone bound to SHBG also serves as a bank to store extra hormone. Only the free, unbound estrogen is active.

To better illustrate the difference between bound (inactive) and unbound (active) estrogen, let's examine the following analogy. A woman has a hundred pieces of her favorite chocolate candy in a bag and decides to eat two pieces of candy. She unwraps two pieces of candy and enjoys it. If she is driving a car, she may decide to unwrap a few pieces and leave them in the bag to make them easily accessible. There are a hundred pieces of candy in a bag but only two to three pieces are unwrapped and accessible. Measuring estrogen and progesterone in the blood reveals how much hormone is in the blood but not how much is accessible to the tissue. Blood measurements reflect the total amount of hormone (candy) present but not how much hormone (candy) is free or unwrapped and accessible.

The normal range of blood estrogen for most labs can vary from 30 milligrams to 500 milligrams. Hormones are very potent. Just a small change in the amount of hormone can cause a major effect. The normal estrogen level range is large because blood levels measure the total amount of hormone, bound and unbound, or wrapped and unwrapped. For instance, a woman who has 400 pieces of candy may have 2-3 pieces of unwrapped candy, while another woman has 50 pieces of candy with 6 pieces unwrapped. Blood tests would show that they both have estrogen levels that fall within the normal range. However, the woman with the lower total amount but more free or unwrapped estrogen would manifest symptoms of estrogen excess.

The salivary glands possess the unique feature of allowing fat-soluble substances to pass from the blood into the saliva. Salivary glands only allow the free, unwrapped portion of estrogen to enter into the saliva. The portion that is bound to the protein carrier cannot enter. This makes saliva an excellent medium to measure the amount of free hormone available to the breast, uterus, brain, and other tissues that are sensitive to sex hormones. This method of testing was discovered in 1959. It took several years to develop methods that could easily and accurately measure free hormones in saliva. Salivary testing is now widely available, and many insurance companies cover the cost. However, this form of testing is still new to most doctors.

Why is Saliva So Important?

Salivary testing can shed light on a lot of problems that have puzzled doctors for many years. The measurement of the total amount of hormone measured by a blood test is meaningless. To make a correct diagnosis, it is necessary to know how much hormone is actually available to the body. Traditional blood tests do not take into account that the amount of bound and unbound sex hormones is constantly changing as carrier protein amounts change.

The body may increase or decrease the amount of estrogen that is free or bound, without affecting the total amount of hormone. Several factors either increase or decrease the amount of carrier protein for estrogen. These factors will determine the total amount of active estrogen available to the tissue.

Let's briefly review some of the factors that effect SHBG (carrier protein) levels.

Weight - Women who are overweight produce less carrier protein. They also produce increased amounts of estrogen in fat tissue. These women have a large amount of available free estrogen. Overweight women are more likely to have irregular bleeding because there is much more free estrogen available than progesterone. They also have an increased risk of breast cancer and uterine cancer. These two cancers are very sensitive to excess estrogen. Overweight women are more likely to have a low fiber diet. A low fiber diet causes estrogen in the bowel to be reabsorbed instead of being eliminated. Approximately 50% of the American population is 20% over their ideal body weight. Therefore, it is likely that a majority of women have increased free estrogen instead of decreased levels of free estrogen.

Overweight women are more likely to be insulin-resistant. They make an excessive amount of insulin, but their body does not respond to it normally. Insulin can drastically lower the estrogen carrier protein (SHBG), which results in increased free estrogen. Women that are diabetic are also at an increased risk for breast and uterine cancer.

Stress - Stress increases the production of a hormone called cortisol. Cortisol decreases the SHBG carrier protein, which in turn increases estrogen levels. In times of stress, women are more likely to have symptoms of estrogen excess.

Diet and Lifestyle - A recent study showed that women who abide by a high fiber and low fat diet have more carrier protein as compared to women with high fat and low fiber diets. The study also showed that an increase in carrier protein, which decreased free estrogen levels, reduced PMS symptoms and pain associated with menses. The women in the study had no significant change in the estrogen levels measured in the blood. Saliva levels were not done on these women.

Exercise - Exercise increases the amount of estrogen carrier protein. Exercise also decreases weight, stress, and insulin levels, all of which effect SHBG levels. The multiple benefits of exercise are associated with a decrease in estrogen excess symptoms.

As you can see, saliva testing is important because blood testing cannot detect changes in SHBG and free estrogen levels. Blood testing only reflects the total amount of estrogen, while salivary testing reflects both the bound and unbound estrogen. Let's review some results of salivary testing and see how it was helpful in diagnosing and monitoring the treatment of the following women.

Case # 1

Hormone	Patient's Salivary Level	Normal Range
DHEA	3 pg/ml (normal)	3-10 pg/ml
Testosterone	9 pg/ml (normal)	8-20 pg/ml
Estrone	75 pg/ml (elevated)	26-64 pg/ml
Estradiol	13pg/ml(premenopausal level)	5-13pg/ml premenopausal
Estriol	<1 pg/ml (low)	4-12 pg/ml
Progesterone	80 pg/ml(low)	100-300 pg/ml

Mary is a slightly obese 54-year-old woman. She had not had a menstrual period for about two years. She complained of fatigue, hot flashes, dry skin, depression, mood swings, and an inability to lose weight. She had experienced symptoms that are associated with menopause.

Her free estradiol level was in the upper range of normal, even though she was obviously menopausal. Her estrone level was elevated due to fat tissue converting androstenedione to estrone. Estrone, in turn, was converted to estradiol, thus increasing her free estradiol to levels found in premenopausal women. Her progesterone level was below normal and her estrogen/progesterone ratio was well below the normal 20 to 1 ratio. She was started on a progesterone cream, which alleviated all of her symptoms.

Case # 2

Hormone	Patient's Salivary Level	Normal
DHEA	16 pg/ml (elevated)	3-10 pg/ml
Testosterone	64 pg/ml (elevated)	8-20 pg/ml
Estrone	>100 pg/ml (elevated)	26-64 pg/ml
Estradiol	26 pg/ml (elevated)	5-13 pg/ml
Estriol	13 pg/ml(elevated)	4-12 pg/ml
Progesterone	<21 pg/ml (low)	100-300 pg/ml

Sarah is another 54-year-old woman who complained of menopausal symptoms. Over the last two years, she complained of hot flashes, decreased sex drive, mood swings, facial hair, and thinning hair. This patient had elevated estrogen and testosterone (male hormone) levels. A possible explanation for these findings is that the male hormones were produced in response to the elevated estrogen levels and low progesterone levels. This also explains why she had male pattern baldness and male pattern facial hair growth.

This patient would have most likely been given estrogen for her menopausal symptoms and testosterone for her decreased libido. However, the saliva test shows she was not deficient in either of these two hormones.

Case # 3

Hormone	Patient's Salivary Level	Normal Range
Estradiol	10 pg/ml (normal)	5-13 pg/ml
Estriol	4 pg/ml (normal)	4-12 pg/ml
Progesterone	<21 pg/ml (low)	100-300 pg/ml

Kim is a 41-year-old woman who was diagnosed with breast cancer in her twenties and underwent surgery to remove one breast. Approximately four years ago, she experienced a recurrence and had the other breast removed, along with chemotherapy and radiation. The chemotherapy and radiation damaged her ovaries and at that time, she began having menopausal symptoms. She was treated with synthetic estrogens and progestins, which made her symptoms worse. She had been prescribed Zoloft® and Synthroid®, but neither relieved her symptoms. When I saw her, she had stopped all medication and reported that her menopausal symptoms were more tolerable without medication.

Surprisingly, her free estradiol level was normal. This may be why additional estrogen increased her symptoms. Her progesterone level was below the measurable range. A progesterone cream was used which increased her progesterone level and improved the patient's menopausal symptoms (hot flashes, mood swings, depression, and bloating).

Case #4

Hormone	Salivary Level	Normal Range
Estradiol	30 pg/ml (elevated)	5-13 pg/ml
Estriol	5 pg/ml (normal)	4-12 pg/ml
Progesterone	87 pg/ml (low)	100-300 pg/ml

Gerri is 46-year-old woman who complained of fatigue, irregular bleeding, severe depression, breast tenderness, bloating, water retention, weight gain, severe mood swings, and anxiety. She had been treated by an endocrinologist for hypothyroidism with Synthroid®, but with little success. She also had multiple D&C's to control her irregular bleeding. Estrogen was recommended, even though her blood estradiol level was normal at 300 pg/ml.

Saliva testing revealed that her free estradiol level was approximately three times the normal level. This patient had already begun using a transdermal (skin) progesterone cream a few days before collecting her saliva, because she was desperate for relief. Even after beginning therapy, her level was still well below what is necessary to balance such a high estradiol level. After three months of transdermal progesterone, this patient reported only occasional vaginal spotting. She was also started on a soy supplement, *Revival ™,* to decrease and block the effects of her elevated estradiol level. On repeat testing, her estradiol level was normal and her estrogen/progesterone ratio was appropriate.

Case #5

Hormone	Patient's Salivary Level	Normal Range
Testosterone	38 pg/ml (elevated)	8-20 pg/ml
Estradiol	10 pg/ml (normal)	5-13 pg/ml
Estriol	5 pg/ml (normal)	4-12 pg/ml
Progesterone	>1000 pg/ml (elevated)	100-300 pg/ml

Lisa is a 52-year-old woman who experienced menopausal symptoms. She started using a progesterone cream twice a day to treat her hot flashes. The hot flashes went away but returned after six months of treatment. Salivary testing revealed extremely high progesterone levels (greater than 1000 pg/ml). The progesterone cream was discontinued for two months. She restarted on a smaller dose every other day. Her symptoms did not return.

Case # 6

Hormone	Patient's Salivary Level	Normal Range
Testosterone	21 pg/ml (elevated)	8-20 pg/ml
Estradiol	13 pg/ml (normal)	5-13 pg/ml
Estriol	10 pg/ml (normal)	4-12 pg/ml
Progesterone	>1000 pg/ml (elevated)	100-300 pg/ml

Julia is a 42-year-old woman who had been on progesterone cream for about a year. Initially, her perimenopausal symptoms greatly improved, but after eight months of treatment, she began experiencing vaginal spotting. Julia began using larger amounts of progesterone cream. Despite increasing the dosage, her initial symptoms returned and she began to experience hair loss.

Salivary testing revealed that Julia had an extremely high level of progesterone. The progesterone cream was discontinued. As her progesterone level decreased, her symptoms improved. Julia had unknowingly recreated a progesterone deficiency because at extremely high levels, progesterone is ineffective. Three months later, another saliva test was done. It revealed the following results:

Hormone	Patient's Salivary Level	Normal Range
Testosterone	15 pg/ml (normal)	8-20 pg/ml
Estradiol	6 pg/ml (normal)	5-13 pg/ml
Estriol	10 pg/ml (normal)	4-12 pg/ml
Progesterone	130pg/ml (normal)	100-300 pg/ml

Julia was much more careful to use the progesterone cream as directed by her physician.

These two cases illustrate the importance of monitoring hormonal levels. Saliva testing allows the physician to monitor the progress of therapy. Even though progesterone has no detrimental side effects, it no longer provides any benefits when it is used excessively.

By using saliva testing, we may be able to end the confusing debate about who needs estrogen. The debate has continued for the past 40 years because there was no accurate method to measure sex hormones. Saliva testing allows doctors to safely prescribe hormone replacement and measure the results of the treatment.

In the following chapters, we will discuss some of the common conditions caused by hormonal imbalances.

Points to Remember

1. **Blood testing is inadequate when used to measure sex steroid hormone levels.**

2. **Hormonal treatment should not be implemented without appropriate testing and documentation of a deficiency.**

3. **Salivary testing is safe and inexpensive.**

4. **Saliva testing is approved by all governmental and laboratory licensing bureaus.**

<u>*Salivary Testing was done by Diagnose-Techs, Inc.</u>

The Washington State Department of Health under the Medical Test Site License program with the biannual renewal licenses Diagnos-Techs. The Washington State License Number is MTS-0327 and the Federal CLIA Number is 50D0630141. The laboratory is licensed and accredited in the specialties of Microbiology, Diagnostic Immunology, and Chemistry. Diagnos-Techs is also accredited by COLA for salivary hormone, GI and other testing. COLA #0011536. Accreditation is awarded to laboratories that apply rigid standards of quality in day-to-day operations.

Chapter 5

Conditions Caused by Estrogen/Progesterone Imbalances

Premenstrual Syndrome

Angela comes to my office for a routine examination. She sits in the exam room looking despondent and desperate. Angela is 35 years old. She reports that her problems began at age 33. Two years ago, she began experiencing heavy menstrual bleeding and cramping along with bloating, swelling and weight gain two weeks prior to her periods. She was prescribed birth control pills to lessen her menstrual cramps and bleeding. She is a nurse, but recently stopped working outside of the home to care for her family. She is concerned about how much rage she has toward her two children at certain times. Her husband is reluctant to come home because of her unpredictable moods. Her marriage has suffered greatly over the last two years. Her husband says that she becomes a different person two weeks before her period. Angela feels like she is tied in a knot. She holds out her hand to illustrate how anxious she is. Her hand is shaking like a leaf. She states that she feels like this for two weeks before her menstrual period. As a result of their marital problems, they started seeing a psychologist. She is on Buspar®, for anxiety, and has been seeing a psychologist over the last year. Her family physician prescribed Buspar®. She and her husband have not noticed any difference in her behavior since she started taking the medication. Angela feels that she is at the end of her rope and desperately wants to know why she feels out of control.

The diagnosis of PMS requires only one of the following symptoms: mild psychological discomfort, bloating and weight gain, breast tenderness, swelling of hands and feet, various aches and pains, poor concentration, sleep disturbance, and change in appetite. The symptom must occur only in the luteal phase (the two weeks prior to the beginning of the menses) of the menstrual cycle, peak shortly before menstruation and cease with the onset of menstrual flow or soon after. This is the criterion for diagnosing PMS according to the Tenth Revision of the International Classification of Diseases. A study done in 1998 by the Woman's Health Research Institute surveyed 220 women who had been given the diagnosis of PMS by a physician. The survey results revealed that on average the women sought treatment for five years before being diagnosed. The women thought that 71% of the physicians were not adequately informed to diagnose and treat them. Twenty three percent used a symptom chart, which is currently the method used to diagnose PMS and only one in four (26%) physicians provided them with helpful treatment.

PMS is a condition that affects over 80% of women in the United States but is undiagnosed by most physicians. Most physicians recognize the 5% of women who suffer from severe PMS. Severe depression, irritability, and mood swings during the last two weeks of the menstrual cycle can interfere with a woman's ability to function at home and work. The cost of this interference can mean career difficulties, loss of income, diminished parenting abilities, and troubled relationships with spouses, and other social acquaintances. The other 75% of women go undiagnosed by the medical establishment. Conventional medicine has not agreed upon a specific cause for PMS, which makes doctors skeptical about its existence. At the same time, PMS is presently so commonplace that it is considered to be a normal occurrence. The treatment of PMS is directed toward eliminating symptoms. Doctors prescribe anxiolytics and antidepressants for anxiety and depression, diuretics for water retention, Motrin® for breast pain and menstrual cramps, and birth control pills for other symptoms such as bleeding. The inadequacy of treatment, the skepticism about the existence of PMS, and the lack of a feasible explanation for PMS symptoms by conventional medicine makes this a subject not readily discussed by most physicians with their patients.

Categories of PMS Symptoms

The symptoms of PMS are grouped in four clusters. The first cluster of symptoms includes tension, anxiety, mood swings and nervousness. Sixty eight to seventy percent of women with PMS complain of these symptoms. There are several studies that show an association between progesterone deficiency and anxiety. In the body, pregnanolone and allopregnanolone are derived from progesterone. These chemicals behave like sedative drugs i.e. Xanax®, Prozac®, Zoloft®, and barbiturates. These drugs are often prescribed for women with PMS. The majority of patients prescribed Prozac® and other selective serotonin re-uptake inhibitors (SSRI's) are women between the ages of 25 to 50. These are also the same age ranges in which women commonly complain about PMS symptoms. A recent study suggests that synthetic SSRI's are helpful in the treatment of PMS because they increase the level of allopregnanolone. In other words, these drugs are mimicking the effect of progesterone. Allopregnanolone binds to GABA receptors, in the brain. Just like any hormone, allopregnanolone must have a receptor that recognizes it in the brain. This GABA receptor also responds to barbiturates and SSRI's, which diminish anxiety and depression.

Studies show that the mental symptoms of PMS are worse in women with markedly elevated estrogen levels during the luteal phase (two weeks prior to menstruation). Remember our discussion about the proper 20 to 1 ratio of estrogen to progesterone? These studies also showed that if the estrogen level exceeded the normal estrogen/progesterone ratio, PMS symptoms increased. Another recent study showed that if higher amounts of SHBG are available to bind estrogen, the symptoms of PMS are lessened. SHBG was increased in this study by dietary changes. Increasing SHBG decreases the amount of active estrogen, which restores the normal estrogen/progesterone ratio.

The second cluster of symptoms that are most often reported are weight gain, abdominal bloating, breast tenderness, and swelling of extremities. Sixty to sixty five percent of women complain of these symptoms. They occur as a result of estrogen's ability to increase aldosterone levels. As mentioned earlier, aldosterone causes fluid retention. Estrogen enhances the effect of aldosterone, while progesterone blocks its effects. If estrogen is elevated and/or progesterone is decreased, aldosterone's influence is increased, which results in fluid retention.

The third group of symptoms includes increased appetite, cravings, headache, and fatigue. These symptoms are identified in approximately 45%-50% of women with PMS. These symptoms are also seen in patients with hypothyroidism or low thyroid hormone levels. Estrogen interferes with the action of thyroid hormone, while progesterone enhances thyroid hormone. Estrogen increases the production of the protein thyroid binding globulin. This protein transports thyroid hormone in the blood. When thyroid hormone is bound to the carrier protein, it becomes inactive. If estrogen levels are elevated, thyroid-binding globulin is elevated and free thyroid hormone is decreased. A low, free thyroid level decreases the body's ability to utilize carbohydrates, fats and proteins. This causes cravings and an increased appetite because the body is unable to effectively use the food consumed. Thyroid hormone has profound effects on the brain. Low thyroid levels can cause depression, weakness, and fatigue.

The final group of symptoms includes depression, confusion, crying, and forgetfulness. Approximately, 36% of women with PMS complain of these symptoms. These symptoms are usually found in the most severe cases of PMS. Neurotransmitters (chemicals that transmit messages within the brain and help control mood) decrease with increasing estrogen levels. The SSRI drugs (Prozac®, Paxil® etc.) that are used for depression increase neurotransmitters called monoamines. Estrogen inhibits the synthesis of monoamines. Endorphins are also a group of compounds made in the brain that normalize or elevate the mood. Estrogen excess in the luteal phase decreases endorphin levels in the brain. Studies have shown that low endorphin levels in the luteal phase are common in women with PMS. Stress decreases endorphin levels and exercise increases endorphin levels. Also, hypothyroidism can cause difficulty with concentration and forgetfulness. Free thyroid hormone directly affects the ability of the brain to utilize the energy needed to perform properly. Stress also decreases the amount of thyroid hormone available.

Premenstrual syndrome (PMS) has been characterized by several symptoms that seem to be related. In conventional medicine, if a group of symptoms seem to be related but there is some uncertainty about the relationship, they are labeled as a syndrome. Because hormones have such a wide range of effects and influence each other, it is confusing and difficult to pinpoint all of their interactions. In addition, when you have ineffective methods to measure hormone and carrier protein levels, it confuses the picture more. Only recently have resources become available that allow conventional doctors to measure free hormone levels, carrier protein levels, and receptors. Today, very few labs and physicians utilize salivary testing to measure free hormone levels. As more studies are being done utilizing more effective laboratory methods, the causes of PMS will move from speculation and theory to documented proof.

Fibrocystic Breast and Breast Pain

Linda is a 35 year-old accountant. Each month prior to her menstrual cycle, she experiences excruciating breast pain. The pain is so bad that she doesn't remove her bra at night. Her breasts swell and are extremely lumpy. Linda's job is very stressful and she drinks large amounts of coffee. Two weeks ago, she found a large lump, the size of a marble, in her right breast. Linda is scared that she might have cancer, so she schedules an appointment with her doctor. A biopsy is performed and fortunately, the lump is benign. Linda is relieved but wants to know how the lump came about and what she can do to keep this from occurring again. Her doctor informs her that the exact cause of her breast disease is unknown. He instructs Linda to avoid caffeine and continue with monthly breast examinations.

Fibrocystic changes in breasts are a relatively common occurrence. The fibrocystic breast feels more granular or lumpy due to small microcysts and thickened connective tissue. Most women complain of breast pain and swelling a week or two before the menstrual cycle. Estrogen causes growth of breast cells. Estrogen can also cause the growth of microcysts and connective tissue in the breast. Studies show that elevated estrogen and low progesterone are found in women with fibrocystic breast. Other studies show that if you correct the estrogen/progesterone ratio imbalance by using a progesterone cream, the breast pain is relieved in 96% of women and the fibrocystic changes are reversed in 86% of women.

It is particularly important to treat fibrocystic changes, if fibroadenomas form and require a biopsy. Fibroadenomas are firm, rubbery, non-tender masses that enlarge slowly over weeks and months. When a fibroadenoma is larger than one inch in diameter or if it is growing rapidly, it should be removed. It is important to remove fibroadenomas to examine them for precancerous cells. If an examination shows that they are present in the fibroadenoma, the patient's risk of breast cancer doubles. A woman who has had more than one biopsy has double the risk of breast cancer versus a woman that has never had a mass in the breast that required biopsy or removal. A woman with fibrocystic breast or a fibroadenoma should consider using progesterone not only to relieve discomfort, but also as a method to possibly prevent breast cancer.

Fibroids

Gloria is a 34-year-old teacher. She is overweight and has tried several diets to lose weight. Over the past several months, her abdomen has become larger. She hasn't missed a period and a home pregnancy test result was negative. Her periods have become prolonged and heavy. She notices that there is a hard mass present in her abdomen. The mass has grown to the point that it is uncomfortable when she walks. Gloria is afraid, but she schedules an appointment. A physical examination reveals that Gloria has a fibroid the size of a grapefruit. She is prescribed Provera® to stop her bleeding. She is scheduled for surgery a few months later. Gloria is unmarried, but she hopes to have children one day. She is reassured that she will be able to have children, but the fibroid is likely to recur. A myomectomy, the surgical removal of a fibroid, is performed, and Gloria goes home with no problems.

Fibroids are non-cancerous growths usually found in the uterus. These growths consist of smooth muscle and fibrous tissue, which start from one abnormal cell. This abnormal cell becomes stimulated and grows more rapidly than the surrounding normal cells. Fibroids can become very large. Large fibroids can cause pelvic pressure, frequent urination, difficulty having bowel movements, and an enlarging abdomen. Fibroids, whether large or small, can cause irregular heavy bleeding, menstrual cramping, and pain during intercourse.

Approximately 25% of reproductive age women develop uterine fibroids. More than 50% of African-American women will develop uterine fibroids. Uterine fibroids are the most common reason why women in the United States undergo a hysterectomy. Hysterectomy (surgical removal of the uterus) or myomectomy (surgical removal of the fibroids only) are two of the most common surgeries performed in U.S. hospitals. The hysterectomy rate in the U.S. is ten times higher than in France.

Could the high rate of fibroids and hysterectomies in women in the U.S. be associated with an estrogen and progesterone imbalance? Medical literature shows that fibroid growth is stimulated by excessive estrogen. Conditions or medications that increase estrogen will stimulate fibroid growth. Conversely, conditions or medications that decrease estrogen will decrease fibroid growth.

Fibroids are more common after ages 30 to 35. During this period of a woman's life, ovulation becomes more irregular. Without regular ovulation there is an inconsistent and inadequate supply of progesterone. There is also an abundance of estrogen. This abundance of estrogen stimulates fibroid growth.

Diet plays a role in fibroid growth. A 1999 study done in Italy showed that fibroid growth was related to the amount of ham and beef that women consumed. Women with a diet high in fruits and vegetables and low in animal fat had fewer fibroids. Animals, particularly cattle and pigs, are given estrogen and other growth hormones to increase their weight prior to slaughter. When women consume the fat of these animals, they consume active hormones, which can stimulate fibroid growth.

After menopause, the total estrogen level is decreased. Fibroid growth also decreases after menopause. A group of drugs called Gonadotropic Releasing Hormone (GNRH) agonists block estrogen production. These drugs shrink fibroids. When the drugs are stopped, the fibroids re-grow.

Progesterone is helpful in decreasing fibroid growth rate and possibly shrinking fibroids. In my clinical experience, progesterone cream has been helpful when the fibroids are small (less than 2 inches in diameter). Large fibroids not only do not respond to progesterone cream, and their growth may be increased with progesterone. It appears that the cells in the fibroid become increasingly abnormal as the fibroid becomes larger.

Other evidence that points to the fact that fibroids are a symptom of an estrogen/progesterone ratio disturbance is that women with fibroids usually have PMS and other symptoms associated with estrogen/progesterone imbalance. Women who have undergone a hysterectomy, but still have their ovaries prior to menopause, do not have monthly menstrual bleeding. However, often they will continue to have monthly premenstrual symptoms. If a woman decides to have the fibroids removed and not her uterus, it is likely the fibroids will recur if she does not begin to make changes to decrease her estrogen exposure.

As you can see, fibroids are a symptom of an estrogen and progesterone imbalance. In order to treat women properly, it is necessary to treat the cause along with the symptom. Women have the ability to make better health choices and avoid becoming a hysterectomy statistic.

Endometriosis

Endometriosis occurs when the cells and tissue from the inner lining of the uterus are somehow transported to areas outside the uterus and begins to grow in abnormal sites. Endometriosis is found in 3% to 10% of reproductive age women and 25% to 35% of infertile women have endometriosis. Painful menstrual periods and pain during intercourse are the most common symptoms of endometriosis.

It is clear that estrogen stimulates the growth of endometriosis. Factors such as diet, lifestyle, and drugs that increase estrogen exposure will increase endometriosis growth.

Factors that decrease estrogen exposure or increase progesterone exposure will decrease endometriosis growth and eliminate mild to moderate endometriosis. Pregnancy is one of the best cures for endometriosis. During the nine months of pregnancy, an abundance of progesterone is produced. Very little estradiol is produced during pregnancy. By decreasing the amount of estrogen present and increasing the amount of progesterone levels, endometriosis is no longer stimulated to grow. Mild to moderate endometriosis is usually eliminated after pregnancy. Breast-feeding, which inhibits menstrual cycles, also decreases endometriosis growth.

Limiting your estrogen exposure can prevent and control endometriosis. We will discuss later how you can limit your estrogen exposure through diet and lifestyle changes.

Points to Remember

1. Most female illnesses that effect premenopausal women are associated with estrogen excess and/or progesterone deficiency.

2. Illnesses caused by estrogen/progesterone ratio disturbances are often misdiagnosed and inadequately treated.

3. Estrogen/progesterone ratio disturbances are most likely to occur between the ages of 35 to 50 years old.

4. Salivary testing is useful in determining whether an estrogen/progesterone imbalance exists.

Chapter 6

Perimenopause: A Time of Transition

Pam

"Doctor, I don't know what is wrong with me. I am 40 years old and for the last two years I feel like everything is falling apart. My menstrual cycles are completely unpredictable. Sometimes, they come every two weeks and at other times they come every two months. My periods can last for two days or two weeks. On occasions, they are so heavy; I am scared I'm going to bleed to death. During the first two days of my cycle, the pain and bleeding is so intense, sometimes I don't go to work. I stay in the house because I'm afraid I may soil my clothes.

I have no energy. I'm gaining weight even though I'm working out three times a week. I can't seem to lose this extra weight. My hips are expanding, I feel like someone is pumping them up with an air hose. I'm miserable the week before I start my menstrual cycle. I begin to bloat and gain weight. I want to stick a pin in myself and drain the fluid from my hands and feet. The people at work kid me about being pregnant because my stomach is so bloated. My breasts don't feel the same. My breasts feel bloated and swollen during this time as well. They become very lumpy and tender. Do you think I need a mammogram or a biopsy? Doctor, I want to be honest with you. During the week before my period, I *crave salt and sugar. I can control myself most of the month, but one week before my period, I'm helpless against my cravings. I have unpredictable mood swings. I feel like Dr. Jekyll and Mr. Hyde. My husband and kids want to move out of the house and stay in a hotel until I turn back into Dr. Jekyll. Unwillingly, I turn into Mr. Hyde. Everything can be going just fine, then my husband walks in the door and I become angry for no apparent reason. He says hello, and I start revisiting unhappy events that happened two years ago and there goes the evening. On other occasions, my children can ask me for a glass of water, and I go on a rampage about how ungrateful they are. Afterwards, I'm depressed because I know that I was out of control but I could not stop myself. I feel so out of control at times. If that's not bad enough, then my migraine headaches come. It's like clockwork, two weeks before my period, the migraines start and I'm helpless and in the bed.*

I really have a wonderful husband and beautiful children. Sometimes, they will find me sitting in my chair, crying. They want to know what's wrong but I can't tell them why I'm crying. I become anxious and tense even though I have nothing to be nervous about. I lay awake at night nervous, unable to go to sleep. I get up the next morning tired, irritable, nervous, depressed and bloated; then my menstrual cycle starts. I don't like feeling this way. My husband thinks I don't love him because I'm not interested in sex anymore. To tell you the truth, I don't feel very sexy most of the month. I really do love my husband, but my sex drive is at an all time low."

Pam's initial complaint was irregular, heavy bleeding. During perimenopause, which usually occurs between age 35 and 45 years old, the menstrual cycle is erratic because ovulation, (egg release) is erratic. Ovulation is the timekeeper and helps to regulate the menstrual cycle. Normally, 14 days after ovulation, a woman begins her menstrual cycle if she has not become pregnant. When a woman does not ovulate the timing of the cycle is disrupted. Between the ages of 18 and 35, the menstrual cycle is usually very predictable and uneventful. A woman is in her peak reproductive years and usually ovulates without interruption. Perimenopausal women are more likely to have cycles in which they do not ovulate (anovulation). When ovulation does not take place, estrogen is produced without an appropriate amount of progesterone. The lining of the uterus grows excessively. Because ovulation has not occurred, the uterus does not know when to shed its excessive lining. This results in heavy erratic menstrual cycles, which disrupt the well being of women, both physically and emotionally.

As a woman ages the cells that mature into eggs also age. In other words, the best eggs ovulate first. The body does not produce new eggs after birth. These aged eggs have more difficulty maturing to a developmental stage in which they can ovulate properly. When ovulation is impaired or absent, progesterone production is diminished or absent. The age of the eggs and frequent anovulatory cycles (without ovulation) cause a wide range of problems. Pregnancy is more difficult, birth defects are more frequent, menstrual cycles are irregular, fibroids appear, the risk of breast cancer increases, bone loss begins, weight increases, and mood swings occur.

Pam's second complaint was low energy and food cravings. Because she is not ovulating, Pam is producing more estrogen than progesterone. Increased estrogen levels affect her thyroid hormone. The problem is not decreased thyroid hormone production, but excess estrogen, which causes the thyroid hormone to be ineffective. Her metabolism slows and her ability to process food into energy is altered. Pam eats properly, sleeps excessively, and exercises but still complains of no energy and weight gain. The sugar and salt cravings are associated with the inability of thyroid hormone to use carbohydrates effectively.

Her bloating and breast tenderness is associated with a lack of progesterone and an abundance of estrogen. Estrogen can over stimulate breast cell growth in the absence of the balancing effect of progesterone. This can cause fibrocystic changes in the breast and breast pain. The swelling of her breast, hands, and feet is the result of a progesterone deficiency and the absence of its diuretic effect (eliminating excess body fluid). The swelling of the tissue around the brain and the nervous system explains the migraine headaches described by Pam.

Decreased progesterone levels caused Pam's mood swings, her anxiousness, depression, and decreased sex drive. Progesterone, as we learned earlier, has a significant influence on the brain's ability to stave off anxiety and depression. Low levels of progesterone and thyroid hormone affect mental concentration. Progesterone may either have a direct effect or an indirect effect on sexual drive. Progesterone is needed to produce testosterone. Testosterone may stimulate sex drive in women. The lack of progesterone along with all of her other symptoms contribute to her decreased sex drive.

If Pam takes the symptom-relief approach, she is faced with the unpleasant task of consuming numerous medications that may cause problems because of their side effects. A birth control pill will decrease and regulate her bleeding. But, it may also increase her chance of blood clot formation. Birth control pills may also cause a zinc imbalance and may accelerate the growth of her fibroids. Most women complain of weight gain on the pill, even though, studies show that there is no significant weight gain as a result of taking birth control pills.

A diuretic, prescribed for bloating, if taken excessively or without the proper replacement of potassium can cause low potassium levels that can lead to life-threatening effects on the heart. Synthoid or thyroid hormone will have no effect on her fatigue and weight gain, because the excess estrogen blocks its function. If too much Synthroid® is prescribed, Pam will begin to experience the symptoms of hyperthyroidism i.e. anxiousness, nervousness and inability to sleep. Now, Pam may need Xanax® to control her anxiety, nervousness and insomnia that have worsened due to Synthroid®.

Prozac® will help with her depression, anxiety and insomnia. However, antidepressants may cause an increase in appetite and weight gain. This is just what Pam needed - more weight. Also, a common side effect of this class of drugs is decreased sex drive. Now, her husband needs an antidepressant.

Most women have increased fibroid growth during perimenopause because of estrogen excess. If nothing is done to correct the imbalance, it is likely that fibroids will grow to a point that surgery is necessary. If Pam had endometriosis, it would worsen during perimenopause. Ovarian cysts occur more frequently during perimenopause. Ovarian cysts develop when a cyst forms and produces an egg, but never ruptures and releases it. It may continue to grow and cause pain at a later time.

The possibility of death as the result of breast cancer is highest during perimenopause. Breast cancer is the leading killer of U.S. women ages 35 to 50. These are also the ages when estrogen production may be greater than progesterone production. There is considerable evidence that estrogen promotes breast cancer growth, whereas progesterone inhibits breast cancer development and growth.

Pam's story is so common. Early in my career as a gynecologist, I was baffled and did not how to help patients like Pam. I too, was guilty of treating the symptoms or, even worse, I would try to change the subject and focus on the things that I could treat. I prescribed birth control pills or progestins like Provera® to control the bleeding. If that failed, surgery was the next option. I dismissed the other symptoms because I had no explanation or treatment for them. Pam and thousands of women face the choice of what to do about their perimenopausal symptoms. By reading this book, you can choose to take steps to balance estrogen and progesterone and regain control of your body, mind, and life.

Points to Remember

1. Perimenopausal symptoms are associated with anovulatory menstrual cycles.

2. Perimenopausal women are more likely to be diagnosed and treated for depression and anxiety.

3. Perimenopausal women are more likely to undergo a gynecological (female) surgical procedure.

4. Saliva testing is important in identifying perimenopausal hormonal imbalances.

Chapter 7

Menopause: A New Beginning

Susan is a 52-year-old lawyer who experienced bleeding, weight gain, bloating, breast tenderness, mood swings, decreased sex drive, fatigue and insomnia during perimenopause. Her periods have stopped, but now she is experiencing hot-flashes. Her hair falls out when she combs it. Hair is growing where she doesn't want it to grow. The Premarin® her doctor prescribed makes her feel worse. Initially, it helped her hot flashes. But, after a couple of months, her bleeding returned. Her breasts are so tender that she can't comfortably wear a bra. It seems as though her depression has worsened. She has gained ten pounds over the past two months that she has taken Premarin®. Susan decides to stop taking her estrogen.

As women transition into and out of the reproductive stage, the estrogen/progesterone ratio is much more subject to instability. The transition into the reproductive stage is called puberty. The transition out of the reproductive stage is called perimenopause. Irregular bleeding, mood swings, weight gain, bloating, painful periods, fibrocystic changes in the breast, and breast pain are common among women during puberty and perimenopause. However, prior to puberty and after perimenopause, the estrogen/progesterone ratio should be irrelevant. During these stages estrogen and progesterone should be very low and stable because there are no cyclic fluctuations of these two hormones caused by ovulation. Menopause should be a time of hormonal stability and balance, but in the United States and Europe this commonly does not occur. This poses the question, "Are women in the U.S. and Europe genetically different from women in other countries?"

Menopausal symptoms are more common in industrialized nations. Women in the United States and Europe complain more of menopausal symptoms than Asian women or women from less industrialized nations. Women in Asia have no vocabulary word in their language for the term "hot flash" because it does not exist in their culture. However, if an Asian woman moves to America or Europe and adopts their diet and lifestyle, the likelihood of menopausal symptoms is equal to an American or European woman. This clearly illustrates that menopausal symptoms are not genetic and unavoidable. In the U.S., menopausal symptoms have become accepted as normal, because so many women in the U.S. seek treatment. Diet, lifestyle, and the environment play a role in menopause. Menopause can be a symptom-free time for women if the right dietary and lifestyle choices are made.

What is Menopause

Menopause usually begins between ages 48 and 52 for women in the United States. Menopause occurs when a woman permanently stops ovulating or producing eggs in the ovaries. During this time, follicles don't need to develop into eggs, the uterine lining does not need to replenish itself, and fat does not need to be stored for procreation. Therefore, less estrogen is necessary. During menopause, the ovary produces little or no estrogen. Ovulation does not occur and progesterone is not produced. Estrogen and progesterone are important throughout a woman's life, but the levels needed for reproduction are not needed during menopause. Enough estrogen can be made by fat, muscle, and skin tissue to maintain the proper function of female tissue, such as the vagina, during menopause.

Estrogens can be found in plants. Plant estrogens found in food sources like soy and flaxseed have the ability to act like estrogen and block estrogen if too much available. Progesterone-like substances can be found in plants, i.e., yams and bloodroot. However, only chasteberry, an herb, has been clinically proven to stimulate progesterone production. The body is unable to produce progesterone outside of the ovary, unlike estrogen.

During menopause, the amount of estrogen and progesterone should decrease proportionately, thereby maintaining the appropriate estrogen/progesterone ratio. If this occurs, women go through menopause without complaints. Menopausal women are often told that their symptoms are caused by an estrogen deficiency, even though the body is able to produce estrogen long after ovulation has ceased.

Menopause is Not a Time of Estrogen Deficiency

Menopause can be diagnosed when a woman no longer has a monthly cycle for a year and has an elevated blood level of FSH. FSH is elevated when a woman stops ovulating or producing an egg. FSH does not reflect the amount of active estrogen in a woman's body, but confirms that a woman has stopped ovulating. Doctors use FSH levels to diagnose menopause. Elevated FSH confirms that progesterone is absent and in no way reflects the amount of estrogen present. Even if blood estrogen levels are decreased during menopause, free and active estrogen levels found in saliva may be normal or high. If you remember, we discussed in previous chapters that the amount of free estrogen is only about 1% to 2% of the total amount found in the blood. The other 98% to 99% is attached to carrier proteins, which transport the hormone in the blood. During menopause, the total amount of estrogen in the blood may be decreased. However, diet, weight, stress, activity level, external estrogen exposure, the ability of the liver and digestive system to process estrogen, and the amount of estrogen carrier proteins can elevate the free estrogen level to a pre-menopausal (before menopause) level. The combination of environmental estrogen exposure and the body's never ending ability to produce estrogen makes it unlikely that estrogen deficiency is the problem in menopause.

Menopause and the Estrogen/Progesterone Ratio

Menopausal symptoms are caused by a disturbance of the estrogen/progesterone ratio. Mood swings can also be traced to progesterone deficiency or estrogen excess. Insomnia is another frequent complaint of women during menopause. It may be attributed to the lack of the calming effects of progesterone and elevated estrogen levels. Replacing progesterone or adding a soy supplement or flaxseed usually improves insomnia.

Many women complain of poor concentration and lapses in memory during menopause. Decreased progesterone and elevated estrogen may interrupt the production of myelin and interfere with brain impulses. Excess estrogen can decrease the amount of free thyroid hormone. As we mentioned earlier, thyroid hormone is necessary to properly metabolize food and convert it into energy. If thyroid hormone is not functioning properly, women will experience weight gain, fatigue, food cravings, and symptoms of low blood sugar. Memory and concentration can be affected. These are all common complaints of menopause.

What may be most disturbing to women are the loss of scalp hair and the growth of facial hair during menopause. The ovary and the adrenal gland can produce testosterone, the male hormone, after menopause. The body produces this hormone to balance estrogen in the absence of progesterone. This results in male pattern baldness and facial hair growth. Replacing progesterone usually reverses this process, initiates growth of scalp hair and stops facial hair growth. Decreasing estrogen levels can also decrease testosterone production.

What About Hot Flashes

Hot flashes are perhaps the number one symptom that motivates women to seek relief during menopause. There is no medically proven cause for hot flashes. The generally accepted explanation is that hot flashes are due to an estrogen deficiency. If you remember from earlier chapters, estrogen has the ability to increase its own receptors. Elevated estrogen levels create more estrogen receptors. As the total estrogen level decreases in menopausal women, the body perceives the decreased level as a deficiency, resulting in hot flashes. Even with a relative decrease in elevated estrogen levels at menopause, estrogen levels can still be elevated, resulting in the other symptoms associated with menopause.

To further understand the cause of hot flashes, let's look at the following illustration. A woman likes a lot of salt and uses it excessively. Her taste buds have become accustomed to excessive salt use. This woman perceives a normal amount of seasoning as being tasteless. Adding more salt to the food remedies the problem. However, we all know that an addiction to salt can be detrimental to the body, resulting in elevated blood pressure, kidney failure, strokes and heart attacks. Pleasure and the avoidance of discomfort motivates most people, therefore the woman continues to add the salt even though it is killing her silently. Similarly, adding more estrogen to a woman who already has estrogen excess is a silent killer. The additional estrogen increases a woman's risk for breast and uterine cancer, stroke and blood clot formation. All of these conditions can lead to premature death. Unfortunately, the addition of the estrogen, like the additional salt, will temporarily make women feel better.

Women in the U.S. have become accustomed to an enormous lifetime exposure to external estrogen. The estrogen level of American women is much higher than that found in women in Asia and other countries that do not suffer with the symptoms of menopause. The production of estrogen made by the ovary decreases during menopause. Progesterone production also decreases. One of progesterone's functions is to control the number of estrogen receptors. The combination of increased estrogen receptor production, secondary to decreased progesterone control, and a decrease in estrogen production results in a perceived relative estrogen deficiency. The body attempts to correct this relative decrease by increasing estrogen production to fill the receptors. The pituitary gland attempts to increase estrogen by producing FSH. The pituitary gland's overzealous attempt to increase estrogen levels stimulates the temperature control center adjacent to it, in the brain, which produces the sensation of a hot flash.

If we can again reflect upon the illustration of the woman with the salt craving, there are a few solutions, which can solve the problem. The woman can simply add more salt. This is synonymous to adding synthetic hormone replacement. As we stated earlier, the level of estrogen that American women are exposed to prior to menopause is excessive. The addition of hormone replacement returns the woman back to abnormally high levels of estrogen. Estrogen replacement is comforting in the short-term and alleviates hot flashes. However, in the long-term, women begin to experience symptoms of excess estrogen again, such as breast tenderness, irregular bleeding, and weight gain. This is probably why only 15% to 25% of women remain on estrogen replacement for more than two years.

Another solution is to use a salt substitute. This satisfies the taste for salt but does not continue to damage the heart and the kidneys. Some substitutes may even prevent or repair damage. Soy and other plant estrogens, along with estriol, a weak estrogen, behave like salt substitutes. These estrogens attach to estrogen receptors and relieve hot flashes. They also maintain female organ function (such as the vagina, breast, bone, and heart) without contributing to estrogen excess. Weak estrogens actually protect the body from stronger estrogens that may stimulate breast or uterine cancers. There are several studies that suggest soy relieves hot flashes, and protects women from breast cancer and osteoporosis. Soy producers have FDA approval to state that it improves cardiovascular health and lowers cholesterol levels.

The third solution is to simply deal with the uncomfortable feeling of not having salt until her taste buds learn to accept food with less salt. This is a long and uncomfortable process for someone accustomed to excessive salt for years. However, she will eventually overcome the craving and the uncomfortable feeling will go away. The same is true for hot flashes as well. Hot flashes will dissipate or fade away in two to five years. The body will eventually adapt to the new estrogen level and stop overreacting to the lower (actually more normal) level of estrogen, and the hot flashes will go away. Again, this is uncomfortable and we are not suggesting that you suffer through it, although some women choose this course of action.   Later in the book, we will discuss treatment options in depth.

The fourth solution is to decrease the number of receptors that need to be filled or satisfied by estrogen. Progesterone has the ability to limit the number of estrogen receptors produced. Estrogen, without the control of progesterone continues to make more estrogen receptors. Progesterone decreases the excessive need for estrogen, produced by increased estrogen receptors, and allows the available estrogen to function normally. There was a recent study done at Temple University in which the researchers treated women complaining of menopausal symptoms with a progesterone skin cream. Progesterone is fat soluble, therefore, the body absorbs it more efficiently through the skin than through the digestive system. Eighty-three percent of these menopausal women reported total relief from their menopausal symptoms. In my clinical practice, I have also found progesterone cream to be effective in treating menopausal symptoms.

Any of these choices are reasonable. Many women are misled into thinking that the only safe option is synthetic hormone replacement. Some women are told that they must take synthetic hormones to prevent heart disease. To date, there is absolutely no evidence that proves that estrogen replacement decreases cardiovascular disease. The FDA specifically restricts the labeling on synthetic estrogen replacement from making the claim that it decreases heart disease. The two largest and most credible studies examining estrogen and heart disease (the HERS and The Women's Health Initiative) actually show that estrogen replacement may increase the risk of heart attack and blood clot formation. The prevention of osteoporosis has also been an indication for estrogen replacement. However, not all women are at risk for osteoporosis. A lot of other factors are involved in the maintenance of strong bones. Estrogen's role in bone health may be overestimated. Hormone replacement for osteoporosis should be prescribed only after salivary testing confirms an estrogen deficiency.

If women are exposed to unbiased truth, we believe they have the ability to choose what is most acceptable to them. There is no single solution for the treatment of menopause. When women are able to understand the origin of their symptoms, they are better able to make choices and initiate changes to improve her health. The chapter on Creating Balance will give you suggestions on how to make menopause a smooth and enjoyable transition.

Points to Remember

1. **Menopause symptoms such as hot flashes, mood swings, and weight gain etc., are not common among women in many other countries.**

2. **Most menopausal women are not estrogen deficient. They have an alteration in the estrogen/progesterone ratio.**

3. **Salivary testing can identify hormonal abnormalities during the menopause and help to determine appropriate treatment recommendations.**

Chapter 8

Osteoporosis: Are Calcium and Estrogen Enough?

Diane is a 62-year-old librarian. She is thin, fair skinned, and exercises very little. Diane also drinks many sodas. Her mother, who recently died, experienced multiple falls and bone fractures. She died, unable to walk and confined to the bed. Diane developed right arm pain and tenderness. She visited her doctor only to find on x-ray that she had a hairline fracture. Diane hasn't had any recent trauma to her arm. She was surprised by the x-ray finding and wanted to know how the fracture could have occurred. She drinks lots of milk, which she thought would make her bones healthy and strong. Her doctor informed her that she might have osteoporosis. Until now, Diane had little knowledge of osteoporosis and wonders if her mother may have had the same condition.

Myths about Osteoporosis

- It is inevitable.
- All women are at risk for osteoporosis.
- Calcium, especially from milk, will prevent osteoporosis.
- Other dietary and behavioral patterns only have a minor effect on osteoporosis.

- Estrogen alone will prevent or reverse osteoporosis.
- Soy and other weaker estrogens have no effect on osteoporosis.
- Premarin is the only estrogen that has an effect on bone loss.
- You have to make a choice between increasing breast cancer risk and preventing osteoporosis.

The word osteoporosis has two root words. The root word "osteo" means bone and "porosis" means porous. Hence, osteoporosis means porous bones. Osteoporosis is a condition in which bone density decreases, resulting in an increased risk for bone fracture. Approximately one million fractures per year are thought to be the result of osteoporosis. The most common fractures are of the vertebrae or backbones, the wrists and the hips. Hip fractures are responsible for approximately fifty thousand deaths annually. Over 50% of Caucasian-American women over the age of 70 will suffer a spinal compression, which is a painful collapse of the bones that form the backbone. It is believed that 25 million Americans have some evidence of osteoporosis.

Osteoporosis can be defined as a disturbance of the delicate balance of bone breakdown and formation. Many women are convinced that they must take estrogen to prevent osteoporosis. While osteoporosis can be a painful, debilitating disease, not all women are at risk for osteoporosis. Estrogen replacement therapy is one treatment for osteoporosis but it does not provide a cure. This chapter will allow you to determine if you are at risk for osteoporosis, and if your risk justifies the use of synthetic estrogens. While synthetic estrogen may be useful for some women, there are other treatment options that can provide the benefits of estrogen replacement without the risks. To help you better understand how you can protect yourself from osteoporosis, we will review bone metabolism, risk factors, prevention, and treatment options for osteoporosis.

How Bones Work

Bone is constantly breaking down and reforming. Bone health is dependent upon mechanical stress (weight bearing), gravity, activity, key nutrients, an intact immune system, and hormonal balance for proper maintenance.

Weight and gravity – When bone is used for weight bearing, the bone can detect its weakest point. By emitting electrical impulses, the bone lays down new strong bone in a weak area and breaks down bone on the opposite side of the weak point, resulting in a uniformly strong bone. This remodeled bone is better able to accommodate the stress of weight. Heavier women are more likely to lay down bone in weak areas than thin women are. Astronauts (men and women) exposed to low or zero gravity for prolonged periods will develop osteoporosis due to the lack of mechanical stress on the bone. This illustrates the importance of weight and gravity in the prevention of osteoporosis in men and women.

Nutrients and Bone – Bone is primarily composed of collagen and hydroxyapatite, which is the mortar that binds the minerals that form bone. Large amounts of collagen make the bones of children flexible and less prone to breakage. Collagen is the substance that forms the ear and is responsible for the elasticity of skin. The majority of bone is made up of hydroxyapatite, which consists of calcium, phosphorous and lesser amounts of several other minerals. Bone also consists of glycoproteins, which are carbohydrates and proteins that re-enforce collagen.

Mineralization – Mineralization is the process during which collagen, glycoproteins and hydroxyapatite (calcium, phosphorous and minerals) come together to form bone. It is necessary to have all three substances available for proper mineralization to take place. This means that the proper type and amount of protein, carbohydrates, calcium, phosphorous and other minerals must be included in your diet for strong healthy bone formation. We will discuss, in detail, the nutrients needed for proper bone health in a later chapter.

Bone Remodeling – Osteoclasts are cells (macrophages) that break down bone. Osteoclasts originate from the immune system. Therefore, an intact immune system is necessary for osteoclast production. Osteoclasts break down the protein, calcium, phosphorous and minerals in bone and release them back into the bloodstream. Osteoblasts are bone builders. They secrete collagen and glycoproteins onto the surface of the bone laying down the glue needed for proper mineralization to take place. The osteoblast buries itself in the bone and becomes a cell called an osteocyte, which helps to maintain the layer of bone it laid down.

Calcium is the most abundant mineral involved in bone mineralization. Calcium is also necessary for many other processes in the body, especially mental function. The bone serves as a calcium bank. Osteoblasts, osteoclasts, hormones, and the immune system regulate how much calcium is deposited or withdrawn from bone. Parathyroid hormone (PTH) is secreted by the parathyroid gland in response to decreased blood calcium levels. PTH decreases the amount of calcium excreted by the kidneys. Osteoblasts direct osteoclasts to break down bone and release calcium into the bloodstream. Cytokines, which are produced by the immune system, are the messengers used by the osteoblast and osteoclasts to stimulate bone remodeling. PTH also activates vitamin D and converts it to calcitrol. Calcitrol increases the absorption of calcium in the small intestine. This increases blood calcium without having to withdraw it from the bone. Parafollicular cells in the thyroid gland secrete calcitonin. **Calcitonin** is secreted when there are increased levels of calcium in the blood. Calcitonin acts directly on bone by decreasing osteoclast activity and increasing osteoblast activity. Calcitonin decreases blood calcium to the normal level and channels the excess calcium towards increasing bone formation.

The Immune System and Bone - Cells within the immune system communicate with cells at other sites through messengers called cytokines. Cytokines regulate osteoblast, osteoclast, vitamin D, estrogen, progesterone, testosterone, and PTH. All of these factors, which effect osteoporosis and calcium balance, are in some way influenced by the action of cytokines and the immune system. Factors that impair the function of the immune system can increase the risk for osteoporosis. **Nitric Oxide** is another chemical messenger that is released by the immune system during periods of infection or inflammation. Small amounts prevent bone breakdown, while large amounts promote bone breakdown. Dietary supplements and synthetic medications that lower nitric oxide improve osteoporosis.

Many dietary supplements that are effective in the treatment of osteoporosis decrease the amount of inflammatory cytokines. Decreasing the amount of inflammatory cytokines inhibits osteoclast from breaking down bone.

As you can see, bone formation and breakdown is very complex. The immune system, endocrine system, kidneys, and intestines along with proper nutrition and exercise all play a role in bone health.

Estrogen, Progesterone and Osteoporosis

Many women are anxious about whether or not they should be on hormone replacement for the prevention of osteoporosis. Women are fearful that if they don't take estrogen and large amounts of calcium, eventually they will become little old ladies with brittle bones and broken hips. From our earlier discussion, you can see that there are many factors involved in maintaining strong healthy bones. Estrogen is only one of many factors that are important in supporting good bone health.

The Facts About Estrogen and Bones: A Review

- Estrogen has not been shown to reduce fractures in women with osteoporosis.

- Bone loss begins at age 35 when estrogen levels are normal or increased.

- Estrogen slows bone loss for only five years immediately following menopause.

- Estrogen only has an effect on osteoclasts. It slows bone breakdown, but has no effect on building new bone.

- Asian women have bone changes that look like osteoporosis on x-ray, but they have significantly fewer fractures. This means that more is involved in preventing fractures than maintaining dense bones on x-ray.

- Women who have anovulatory menstrual cycles or who no longer ovulate have increased risk of osteoporosis. Elevated estrogen levels are associated with these conditions.

- Women who miss more than 50% of their menses have 31% more bone loss than women who miss less than 50% of their menses. Women who miss menses are more likely to be low in progesterone not estrogen. Estrogen production does not depend upon ovulation. Estrogen is made in fat tissue and by the follicular cyst prior to ovulation.

- Estrogen has no effect on women who develop osteoporosis from steroid use. This implies that other mechanisms are involved other than estrogen. Steroids attach to the progesterone receptor on osteoblasts, which build bone. This further supports the fact that progesterone has a role in bone formation.

- While estrogen has received most of the attention in the prevention of osteoporosis, just as much unpublicized, credible data shows that several other factors need to be addressed as well.

Other facts about bone health include:

- Progesterone and testosterone stimulates osteoblasts, which are involved in bone growth.

- Women with short cycles (less than 21 days) have less dense bones than women with normal length menstrual cycles (26 days or more). Shorter cycles are usually anovulatory cycles.

- Cortisol, a hormone associated with chronic stress, may play a role in osteoporosis. Stress negatively affects the immune system and can block the actions of osteoblasts, which are bone-building cells.

- Steroids such as prednisone prevent osteoblasts from building bone, thus causing osteoporosis. Progesterone prevents this steroid effect on bone.

- Exercise and activity prior to age 35 builds bone and prevents osteoporosis more effectively than estrogen.

- Exercise has been shown to increase bone mineral density by 3.5% in the bones of the back.

- A diet rich in fruits and vegetables is associated with decreased osteoporosis.

- Calcium balance is more important than calcium intake.

- Calcium is lost with excessive animal protein intake.

- Calcium is lost with excessive carbonated cola consumption. They contain phosphorus, which facilitates calcium loss.

Do I really need to worry about osteoporosis?

To answer this question, let's examine some risk factors and see if you are at risk for osteoporosis.

Risks for Osteoporosis

Women

Caucasian, especially of Northern European descent

Family history

Low body weight

Sedentary lifestyle

Smoking and alcohol use

Steroid use

Other risk factors include:

- **Frequent missed periods or anovulatory cycles**
- **Decreased exercise or physical activity during teenage years**
- **Decreased exposure to sunlight**
- **Excessive carbonated drinks and caffeine consumption**
- **Excessive consumption of animal protein**

Women - It is well established that women are much more likely to develop osteoporosis than men. This may be due to a host of factors, including smaller body mass, genetic factors, and hormonal imbalance. Bone metabolism is optimally maintained when both estrogen and progesterone are available in their appropriate ratio of 20 to 1. Women with normal menses before age 35 are not at an increased risk for osteoporosis. Women with abnormal or irregular menses and diminished progesterone levels prior to age 35 have less bone density than women with normal menses. Bone loss begins at age 35 when progesterone usually declines, and estrogen levels are normal or high. Women with normal estrogen/progesterone ratios during the postmenopausal period should have a decreased risk of osteoporosis. Postmenopausal women with normal estrogen/progesterone ratios have proportional decreases of progesterone and estrogen, thereby maintaining the 20 to 1 ratio. Studies are being conducted to substantiate whether this can be proven clinically.

Caucasian Women and Family History - These two risk factors indicate that a genetic component exists in osteoporosis. Caucasian women of North European origin are at an increased risk for osteoporosis. While there is nothing you can do about your genetic makeup, avoiding controllable risk factors may determine whether you develop osteoporosis. African American women and other non-

Caucasian races are generally not at high risk for osteoporosis. Non-Caucasian fair skinned women who have several risk factors may need to be screened for osteoporosis. After menopause, Asian women generally have decreased bone mass but have fewer fractures. The architecture of Asian women's bones may be stronger because of some genetic or environmental factor. This reiterates the point that we do not know all the factors that contribute to the development of osteoporosis and bone fractures.

Low Body Weight - Women with low body weight are at an increased risk for osteoporosis because there is less stress on the bone, which leads to a decrease in bone remodeling and rebuilding. Earlier, we discussed how the stress of weight, whether it is in the form of body weight or weight-bearing exercise, causes stress on the bone. The bone responds to the stress by remodeling and laying down more bone to strengthen itself. Astronauts in low or no gravity environments for extended periods of time, experience significant bone loss due to decreased bone stress. Women who are 20% or more above their ideal body weight are not at great risk for osteoporosis. Over 60% of women in the U.S. are 20% above their ideal body weight. Women with low body weight should participate in weight bearing exercises at least three times a week.

Sedentary lifestyle - A sedentary lifestyle also decreases mechanical stress on bones. The phrase "If you don't use it, you will lose it" applies here. Women who are confined to wheelchairs or to the bed will develop some degree of osteoporosis. It is especially important to be active prior to age 35. This is when bone mass is actively accumulated. Active teenagers and young adults have higher peak bone mass at age 35 and are less affected by any bone loss after age 35.

Smoking - Smoking has direct and indirect negative effects on bone health. Smoking damages the liver and speeds up the metabolism of steroid hormones, such as estrogen, progesterone, and testosterone. All of these hormones are involved in maintaining healthy bones. Smokers are more likely to be deficient in vitamins and minerals that are essential in building bone. Smokers are also more likely to have a lower activity level because of the detrimental effect that smoking has on the lungs. Smoking negatively affects the immune system, which is vitally important in maintaining healthy bones.

Alcohol - Excessive alcohol use increases fractures because alcoholics are more likely to fall. Alcoholics are also more likely to eat a diet deficient in proteins, vitamins and nutrients that are important for bone building. Alcoholics are usually exposed to excessive estrogen levels because of the inability of the alcoholic's liver to eliminate estrogen from the body.

Steroid use - Women and men who have been treated with steroids for a long period of time are at an increased risk for osteoporosis. Steroids like Prednisone are used to treat chronic asthma and autoimmune disorders such as lupus. Steroids are used to blunt or deactivate the immune system. By blunting the immune system, steroids decrease the positive effect of cytokines (messengers) on the bone. Steroids also directly affect the osteoblast. These steroids can bind the progesterone receptor on the osteoblast, which prevents the osteoblast from building bone.

Calcium Imbalance - Calcium is especially important to the proper maintenance of bone. Most women are told that they need to increase their calcium consumption if they want to maintain strong bones. Calcium levels are controlled not only by how much calcium is consumed, but also by how much is excreted. Americans have to consume more calcium because poor dietary habits cause the elimination of excessive amounts of calcium in the urine. Not every woman has a calcium deficiency. If a woman eats foods that are rich in calcium and avoids large amounts of meats and carbonated beverages, it is unlikely that she will need to take calcium supplements.

Carbonated sodas and caffeine - The phosphorous contained in carbonated sodas can directly bind to calcium in the bone and cause it to be excreted into the urine. Caffeine, which is found in most colas, carbonated drinks, and coffee, causes the following to occur:

- Increases the excretion of calcium in the urine
- Decreases blood calcium levels
- Causes calcium to be removed from the bone

Recent studies show that teenagers who consume higher amounts of carbonated sodas have more bone fractures than teenagers who consume less carbonated sodas. This is very alarming. We may be witnessing the beginning of an osteoporosis epidemic as a result of our growing obsession with carbonated drinks.

Animal protein - Protein is essential in building bone. Too little protein definitely contributes to the development of osteoporosis. People who do not consume enough protein are at a high risk for osteoporosis. The recommended daily allowance of protein per day is 63 grams. It is not unusual for the typical American to consume more than 100 grams a day of animal protein. Protein derived from animal sources prompts the body to excrete more calcium. Raising the consumption of animal protein from 50 grams to 150 grams doubles calcium excretion. The type of protein that a woman consumes is important. Plant-based protein found in green leafy vegetables and beans or legumes do not increase calcium excretion or bone loss. Women who adhere to a predominantly plant-based diet have an average of 18% bone loss by age 80. Women who consume animal protein have an average of 35% bone loss by age 80. While dietary supplements have been shown to decrease bone loss, the most effective method to obtain key vitamins and minerals is by increasing your consumption of fruits and vegetables.

It is important to note that while Americans don't consume an adequate amount of calcium, it is also true that most Americans excrete an excessive amount of calcium. The American habit of eating meat with every meal and very few green, leafy vegetables that are high in calcium contributes to our calcium imbalance. Our teenagers are being raised on a fast food diet of hamburgers, fries, pizza, and sodas. This fast food diet is very detrimental to young adult bone health at a time when bone formation should be at its maximum level. Until women are willing to make dietary changes, osteoporosis is going to continue to be a significant problem in America.

The prevention of osteoporosis is not as simple as prescribing estrogen and increasing calcium intake. Several studies show that estrogen is only useful in high-risk women. The FDA has approved estrogen use only in high-risk women. Low-risk women do not need to take estrogen replacement to prevent osteoporosis. Objective testing by saliva testing can be used to determine if a woman is estrogen-deficient and at risk for osteoporosis.

It is fortunate that there are identifiable and controllable risk factors for osteoporosis. Women can take actions to eliminate or decrease the effect of these risk factors. By making wiser choices, women can protect themselves from osteoporosis, which is not an inevitable disease.

Points to Remember

1. **Osteoporosis is preventable.**
2. **Not all women are at risk for osteoporosis.**
3. **Progesterone deficiencies before and after menopause may play a role in the development of osteoporosis.**
4. **Estrogen is not a cure for osteoporosis.**
5. **Good dietary habits are crucial to maintaining proper bone health.**

Chapter 9

Breast Cancer: Stop Living in Fear

Cathy is a 31-year-old woman who comes to see her doctor for a mammogram. She has had unusual breast pain around her nipple, for the last month. She also has noticed a discharge from her left breast when she squeezes it. The discharge is clear and only discharges when she squeezes her breast. She performs self-breast exams on a regular basis, but she is worried that she doesn't know what she is doing and might have breast cancer. Suddenly, Cathy cries out, " I just don't want to die!" and begins to cry, uncontrollably.

Cathy begins to tell her doctor why she is so anxious and fearful. "My closest friend at work just died of breast cancer. She was 31! I had known her for 10 years. She was not any different from me. She made regular visits to the doctor. She checked her breast and found a small lump two years ago, and now she is dead. I can't go to sleep at night because I keep thinking about how her husband and children must feel without a wife and mother. I remember how depressed my friend was when she had to endure the surgery, the chemotherapy, losing her hair, and feeling weak and sick after each dose of chemotherapy. I also remember how brave she was close to the end of her life. She tried to be strong for her family and friends. She was optimistic that she could lick this thing, but she didn't."

Her doctor consoles her and alleviates some of Cathy's fear by ordering a mammogram. However, because the breast tissue in women before age 35 is so dense, it will be difficult to identify breast cancer by mammogram. Cathy's fear is legitimate because young women (age less than 50) are more likely to die from breast cancer than any other cause, including heart disease. Mammograms are designed for early detection - not prevention. Cathy wants to know what placed her friend at risk for breast cancer and how she can decrease her risk for breast cancer.

No subject provokes more fear in women than the thought of developing breast cancer. This diagnosis can change a woman's life forever. Women with breast cancer are faced with the fear of losing their breasts, sexuality, and possibly their lives. Regardless of whether they have breast cancer that is easily treated or cancer that is in a very advanced stage, women who have breast cancer battle with the fear of premature death on a daily basis. This fear of breast cancer is understandable. American women have a 1 in 8 chance of developing breast cancer in their lifetime. In Asia, parts of Africa and in other less developed countries, the risk of breast cancer is as low as 1 in 100. A recent study in the New England Journal of Medicine studied 90,000 sets of twins and found that breast cancer could only be considered inherited in 27% of the cases. This means that 73% of the breast cancer cases were caused by environmental factors. Studies also show that when a woman moves from a low-risk country to a high-risk country like the United States or Europe, the woman develops the risk of breast cancer associated with the high-risk country.

A better understanding of how breast cancer develops, what makes it grow, and lifestyle changes that prevent breast cancer, is important if women are going to win the battle against breast cancer.

Estrogen, Progesterone and the Normal Breast

As with other female organs, estrogen and progesterone are primarily responsible for normal breast development and health. Estrogen has a major influence on breast growth during puberty. Estrogen stimulates the growth of breast ducts, and progesterone influences the growth of the milk-producing glands called the alveoli. Other hormones, especially prolactin, are required for full breast development. Pregnancy completes the development of the breast. The influence of increased levels of prolactin, progesterone, and estrogen (specifically estriol) during pregnancy matures the breast cell completely.

Studies have shown that estrogen increases the rate at which cells replicate or increase in number. During cell replication, a cell makes copies of itself. The information contained in the cell will be copied tens or hundreds of times. Progesterone has been shown to decrease the rate of replication and promote cell maturation. It is important for breast cells to mature and develop if they are to function properly. The increased amount of progesterone produced during pregnancy is important in the maturation of the breast cell.

Estrogen and progesterone, when present in their proper ratio, create healthy breasts. With each menstrual cycle, estrogen is initially produced to increase the number of breast cells. After ovulation occurs, progesterone stimulates these cells to develop and mature. Progesterone is also involved in promoting normal cell death. Cells have a normal life span that is programmed in their DNA. This programmed cell death is called apoptosis. Without regular cell death, overcrowding and chaotic cells lead to breast cancer.

What is Breast Cancer?

Cancer develops when there is an uncontrollable growth of cells. These cells are immature and behave in an uncharacteristic manner. Each cell in your body has the information (DNA) required to carry out normal cell function. The information in the breast cell DNA is the same as the information in a liver, brain or heart cell. A very delicate and intricate process determines which information is expressed in a particular cell. The information that controls the expression of a gene (a segment the DNA) is found in the DNA. The information in the DNA is very precise but vulnerable. One small blemish in the DNA can cause enormous problems.

The current theory explaining the development of cancer involves two events. DNA is damaged by free radicals. This is followed by the replication of cells containing the damaged DNA. Free radicals are oxygen molecules that are missing an electron. Free radicals are produced from fat metabolism, solar and ionizing radiation, cigarette-smoke exposure, pollutants, heavy metals, food additives, organic solvents, and pesticides. It is believed that these environmental factors are the major contributors to the high rate of breast cancer in America.

When DNA damage occurs, cells have the ability to repair the majority of the damage. Antioxidants found in foods or supplements can add an electron to the free radical oxygen molecule, thereby restoring it to a normal, safe oxygen molecule thus preventing further damage. Fortunately, most of these damaged cells are dormant and never replicate.

Cancer develops when these damaged cells:

1. **Replicate rapidly**
2. **Lose their identity**
3. **Live longer**

Estrogen, Progesterone and Breast Cancer

Estrogen stimulates the production of new, immature cells. These new cells are dependent upon progesterone for development into mature cells. Immature breast cells are more vulnerable to DNA damage from free radicals. To illustrate the point better, let's look at the following analogy. Children and teenagers are more likely to be swayed by outside influences that can damage their future development and prevent them from carrying out their intended purpose in life. On the other hand, it is very hard to persuade a mature adult who understands his or her purpose and identity to engage in uncharacteristic behavior. Immature breast cells, like children and teenagers, are easily influenced by outside influences.

It is obvious that while estrogen may not initiate the changes that result in breast cancer, estrogen plays a significant role in promoting the growth of breast cancer. Estrogen stimulates normal and abnormal breast cells to grow. **When a damaged breast cell receives the message to grow from estrogen, it begins to:**

1. **Replicate rapidly**
2. **Lose its identity because progesterone is unable to mature the cell**
3. **Live longer in the absence of appropriate amounts of progesterone**

Risk Factors for Breast Cancer: Are Estrogen and Progesterone Involved?

The Major Risk factors for Breast Cancer are:

1. Starting menses younger than 12 years old
2. Menopause after age 55
3. Greater than age 30 at the time of first live birth
4. A lump in the breast requiring biopsy
5. Family history of breast cancer
6. Obesity
7. Alcohol use
8. Estrogen replacement therapy

As the number of risk factors increase so does your risk of breast cancer.

Women who start their menses at an age less than twelve are exposed to more menstrual cycles than women who start later. With each cycle comes estrogen exposure and thus stimulation of breast cells. Menstrual cycles, which begin early in a woman's life, are usually void of ovulation. This results in little or no production of progesterone. The absence of progesterone leaves immature breast cells vulnerable to damage from environmental factors.

Late menopause results in the same scenario. The more menstrual cycles woman experiences, the more opportunity there is for non-ovulatory cycles. A woman who experiences late menopause has a prolonged perimenopausal period. During perimenopause, the estrogen/progesterone ratio becomes less stable. This allows estrogen to strongly influence the growth of breast cells. When estrogen influences an abnormal cell to grow, breast cancer is the result.

Earlier in this chapter, it was mentioned that pregnancy completely develops the breast cell. The earlier in life the pregnancy occurs, the greater the protection from breast cancer. Women who have their first live birth by age 18 have one-third the risk of breast cancer than women who have their first pregnancy after age 30. The mature breast cell is less vulnerable to damage and the effects of estrogen, and is less likely to begin replicating again under the influence of estrogen.

Benign (non-cancerous) breast disease requiring a biopsy increases the risk of breast cancer. Fibrocystic changes that never require a biopsy have no influence on breast cancer rates. If a woman has one biopsy, her risk of breast cancer increases by 50%. If two of a woman's biopsies are benign, or if one of her biopsies shows rapidly dividing cells, her risk of breast cancer doubles. A biopsy that yields slightly abnormal and rapidly growing cells increases the breast cancer risk by four times.

Studies show that the administration of estrogen can increase the rate of breast cell replication up to 200 times the normal rate. These same studies show that if progesterone was administered along with estrogen, the cell replication rate did not increase. This proves that progesterone can override and regulate the influence of estrogen on breast cells. As mentioned earlier in the book, a progesterone deficiency is often found in women with non-cancerous breast changes. It has also been shown that progesterone, given in the form of a skin cream, can reverse fibrocystic breast changes in 85% of mild cases.

Obesity increases breast cancer risk. Obese women make a large amount of estrone in fat tissue. Estrone may negatively influence the breast more than the other two estrogens, estradiol and estriol. Free radicals are produced by the metabolism of fat; therefore, obese women produce more free radicals. Fat tissue stores environmental toxins that may initiate cancer. Non-diabetic obese women produce a lot of insulin. Insulin stimulates the growth of cells and makes breast cells more sensitive to estrogen. Increased fat tissue and weight increases the amount of free estrogen available by decreasing the amount of SHBG. Obese women are, therefore, at an increased risk of breast and uterine cancer because of increased free estrogen levels.

Alcohol use increases breast cancer risk by decreasing the liver's ability to eliminate estrogen. The liver and the large intestines are the primary sites of estrogen elimination. Alcohol damages the liver, making it inefficient in metabolizing estrogen. Most alcoholics have very poor diets. Their diet usually lacks vitamins and nutrients, such as vitamin B and E, which the liver needs to metabolize estrogen. The large intestine needs fiber to help eliminate estrogen. Fiber is usually not a large part of an alcoholic's diet. The risk of breast cancer increases by 70% in women who are moderate to heavy drinkers (two to four drinks a day). However, women who drink a glass of wine a day do not appear to have an increased risk.

Estrogen Replacement Therapy and Breast Cancer

Nothing has been debated more among gynecologists than the question; "Does estrogen replacement cause breast cancer?" All of the risk factors for breast cancer are associated with increased estrogen levels and/or decreased progesterone levels. Most physicians are very quick to stop estrogen replacement if a mammogram suggests any abnormal growth. There are over a hundred studies that show that estrogen promotes the growth of breast cancer. But, an equal number of studies exist that show no effect. You might ask, which studies are correct?

The answer seems to depend upon how long a woman has been taking estrogen. The Director of Analytical Epidemiology at the National Cancer Institute, wrote an article that discussed her conclusion after surveying all of the articles written on estrogen replacement and breast cancer. **Her conclusion was that taking estrogen replacement for more than five years increases a**

woman's risk of breast cancer by 20%. This conclusion explains why there is so much confusion and disagreement about the studies on breast cancer. Studies that showed no effect of estrogen on breast cancer rates included a mixture of women that had taken estrogen for various lengths of time. These studies included women who had taken estrogen for less than four years. If women who had taken estrogen for one year were included with women who had taken estrogen for ten years, the results would cancel each other out. Most studies that have observed women with greater than five years of estrogen replacement therapy revealed an increased risk of breast cancer. The good news is that women who discontinue the use of estrogen return to their normal risk level after two years. The risk returns to normal even if a woman has taken estrogen for more than four years.

Current evidence does not support the use of long-term estrogen replacement therapy. Estrogen replacement works very well to relieve hot flashes and other symptoms associated with menopause on a short-term basis. However, its long-term benefit has not been proven. As we discussed earlier in our chapter on osteoporosis, estrogen may only play a small role in prevention of fractures. The long-term risk of estrogen replacement has been established. If you do choose to take synthetic estrogen replacement, you should take it for no longer than four years. During that four-year period, we suggest that you incorporate diet and lifestyle changes, which will be covered in depth in Chapter 11, Creating a Balance.

Progesterone, Progestins and Breast Cancer

The effect of progesterone and progestins on the breasts continues to be confusing to most doctors. The confusion is fueled by the fact that these two terms are used interchangeably to describe progesterone. As you now know, these substances are chemically different.

Progestins are synthetic or manmade substances that make the lining of the uterus produce secretory cells. Secretory cells normally result from the production of progesterone after ovulation. Progestins were developed to counteract the effect of estrogen replacement on the uterus. With the implementation of estrogen replacement, which began in the 1960's, the rate of uterine cancer increased drastically. This was obviously a serious side effect of synthetic estrogen replacement.

Oral progesterone could not be used because the liver destroys it when taken by mouth. Progestins, which are not destroyed by the liver, were developed to prevent endometrial cancer in women on estrogen replacement.

Progestins were designed to mimic the effect of progesterone on the endometrium. Progestins solved the problem of uterine cancer, but they are unable to perform the other functions of progesterone that are important to female health.

Studies show that progesterone also has a protective effect on breast tissue. A 1981 study performed at Johns Hopkins University scrutinized women in their infertility clinic who had symptoms of progesterone deficiency. The study compared this group of women to women with non-hormonal causes of infertility. The study found that the women with a progesterone deficiency had a premenopausal rate of breast cancer five times higher than the group of women without progesterone deficiency. The study also showed that the women with progesterone deficiency were ten times more likely to die from any cancer as compared to the other group of women.

No other differences existed between the two groups' risk factors. In other words, the only risk factor that was different in the two groups was the amount of progesterone they produced. This finding confirmed that the presence of progesterone diminishes the rate of breast cancer in young women. This finding is also of great importance because breast cancers in young women are usually more aggressive and more likely to lead to death. Breast cancer is the leading cause of death in women younger than age 55. As we discussed earlier, women between the ages of 35 and 50 are more likely to experience anovulatory cycles. This leads to a relative progesterone deficiency, thus creating conditions similar to the group of women in the study above.

Studies performed using laboratory breast cancer cells have shown that progesterone promotes normal cell death in breast cancer cells. In one study, progesterone was applied to a group of breast cancer cells. Subsequently, the cells returned to a normal life span. The other breast cancer cells that did not receive progesterone had a prolonged, abnormal life span.

Studies involving patients with abnormal breast cells have shown favorable results as well. A 1995 study attempted to show the effect of adding progesterone to the breast. The study included women that were scheduled for a breast biopsy to remove a lump. One group of women applied a progesterone cream to the breast for ten days prior to surgery. Another group applied estrogen and progesterone to the breast. Another group applied estrogen only and the last group did nothing.

The study showed that applying a progesterone cream decreased the number of replicating cells in the breast by three times as compared to the group that did nothing. Compared to the group that applied estrogen to the breast, it lowered the amount of replicating cells five times.

What may be most important is that in the group that applied estrogen and progesterone, the cell replication rate was equal to the group that did nothing.

This means that progesterone can counteract the effects of excess estrogen. Excess estrogen is believed to be the culprit in the majority of cases of American women who develop breast cancer, especially at the perimenopausal age when breast cancer is the most deadly.

A study done in France looked at over 1,100 women with fibrocystic breasts. Fifty-eight per cent of the women were using a progesterone cream. The women using the cream had a 20% decreased risk of breast cancer. This study did not have enough women involved and was not extended for a long enough period of time to prove that progesterone prevents breast cancer. However, it did show that progesterone does not seem to increase the risk of breast cancer.

A study that was published in the Journal of the American Medical Association in January of 2000 reported that women on estrogen replacement alone had a 20% increased risk of breast cancer after four years of use. The study also showed that women on estrogen and progestin therapy had a 40% increased risk of breast cancer. This finding surprised the majority of the medical community.

For those who understand the difference between progesterone and progestins, the results of the study were logical. Progestins displace progesterone from progesterone receptors. This prevents progesterone from having a protective effect on the breast cell. Progesterone is unable to mature the breast cell, which makes the cell more vulnerable to environmental factors and increases the risk of breast cancer.

Because there is confusion in the medical community about the differences between progesterone and progestins, women are bombarded by conflicting information regarding the benefits of progesterone. The limited use of progestins has its place, but there are greater benefits from progesterone if used correctly.

Breast Cancer: The Final Word

The cure and prevention of breast cancer is multi-faceted. There is significant evidence that there are some controllable risk factors involved in breast cancer. We believe that the evidence presented overwhelmingly confirms that estrogen has a negative influence on the breast cells in the absence of adequate amounts of progesterone. This negative influence may be expressed as breast pain, tenderness and non-cancerous and cancerous breast growths. Making the decision to minimize your risk for breast cancer by decreasing your estrogen exposure is imperative if you are going to win the battle over breast cancer. (see page 130 for the outcome of the Women's Health Initiative).

Points to Remember
1. **Cancer is an uncontrolled growth of damaged cells.**
2. **Estrogen stimulates growth.**
3. **Risk factors for breast cancer are associated with an increase in estrogen exposure and or decreased progesterone production.**
4. **The use of synthetic hormone replacement for more than four years increases breast cancer risk by 20 to 40%.**
5. **Diet and lifestyle play important roles in the development and prevention of breast cancer.**
6. **Finally, get a saliva test to determine if you have elevated estrogen levels or decreased progesterone levels, which increases your risk for breast cancer.**

The Women's Health Initiative

The Women's Health Initiative (WHI) was a ten-year study designed by the National Institute of Health to compare various treatments for menopausal symptoms. One arm of the study observed the effects of diet and lifestyle changes, another arm prescribed Premarin® alone and the third arm of the study prescribed Premarin® and Provera®. The medical community, pharmaceutical industry and general public were greatly anticipating the outcome of the study. The medical community and pharmaceutical industry were convinced that this comprehensive non-biased study would put to rest all of the doubts about the health benefits of long term hormone replacement therapy. The general public wanted to end the confusion surrounding the issue of hormone replacement.

The findings of the WHI were specific to women who were prescribed Premarin® and Provera®. The findings are not to be extrapolated to other therapies. None of the women involved in the study were tested to determine if they needed hormone replacement. They were given a therapy based on age, symptoms and a FSH test, which does not correlate with estrogen levels but only determines if a woman is menopausal.

The WHI was discontinued after 5 years because of the following findings:

1. Breast cancer risk was increased by 26%

2. Heart disease risk was increased by 29%

3. Stroke risk was increased by 41%

4. Pulmonary emboli or lung blood clots were increased by 213%

After the study was halted, more intense review of the data revealed:

5. Abnormal mammograms increased by 120,000 a year from Premarin and Provera use.

6. Breast cancer risk increased after 1 year of use and the cancers were more advanced when diagnosed.

7. Dementia or senility was increased in women over 65 using Premarin and Provera.

8. Premarin and Provera did not improve a woman's quality of life.

Forty two per cent of the participants in the Premarin and Provera arm of the study dropped out of the study. Therefore, it was extrapolated that the risk would have been higher if all of the women had completed the study. A recent study in Britain, which included a million women, found that the risk of breast cancer was, increased by 66% for woman using Premarin and Provera further supporting the findings of the WHI. The take home message of the outcome of the WHI study is; **the risks associated with the use of Premarin and Provera clearly outweigh their benefit (relief of hot flashes).**

Chapter 10

Heart Disease Prevention and Estrogen

Brenda is a 41-year-old dentist. She is really concerned about all the information in the news concerning estrogen and breast cancer. Brenda has read that more women die of cardiovascular disease than breast cancer. The literature reports that estrogen lowers cholesterol levels and therefore lowers the risk for heart disease. Women who take estrogen have fewer heart attacks than women who don't take estrogen. Brenda feels torn. She wants to decrease her risk of heart disease, but she does not want to increase her risk of breast cancer.

What should Brenda do? Many women are faced with Brenda's dilemma each day. Should I take estrogen to prevent heart disease, even though it might increase my risk of breast cancer?

Conventional medicine surmised that estrogen prevented heart disease when it discovered that estrogen had the effect of lowering cholesterol. Estrogen lowers the LDL cholesterol, which is thought to have significant effect on heart disease. The second piece of information that convinced doctors that estrogen prevented heart disease was the Nurses Health Study. This study followed several thousand nurses over several years and scrutinized their lifestyles and health outcomes. The Nurses Health Study showed that the nurses who took estrogen during their lifetime had fewer heart attacks than the nurses who had not taken estrogen.

The Nurses Health Study was an observational study. This means that a select group of people were observed for differences, and conclusions were drawn from the observations. The problem with study was that the observers could not randomize and control for other factors that may have influenced their observations. There are several lifestyle and dietary factors that have been proven to lower the risk of heart disease and even reverse heart disease. An ideal study is a randomized, controlled study in which neither the patients nor the observer knows what is being observed. The Nurses Health study revealed the influence of "the healthy user effect." Women who use estrogen replacement are more likely to be more health-conscious than women who do not use estrogen replacement. They are more likely to engage in behaviors, which would have a positive effect on their health. Observational studies are uncontrolled and are influenced by many factors such as exercising, healthy dietary habits, smoking, weight, stress, etc. The drawback of observational studies is that the observer is never quite sure if the outcome observed is actually caused by what is being observed. Therefore, it is hard to draw definitive conclusions from these studies.

The FDA approves what can be said about estrogen replacement and only allows proven facts about estrogen replacement to be included in the package insert. **The package insert for estrogen replacement includes the following statement:**

> **"A causal relationship between estrogen replacement and prevention of cardiovascular disease in postmenopausal women has not been proven."**

There are two important, large studies, which have used the randomized, controlled method to examine the relationship between cardiovascular disease and estrogen replacement. The first study, The Heart Estrogen Replacement Study (HERS) explored the use of estrogen in postmenopausal women who had a previous heart attack. Observational studies had shown that estrogen prevented heart attack. Therefore, it was logical that estrogen would be beneficial to women who had had a heart attack. The HERS study found that women who took estrogen were more likely to have a fatal heart attack than women who had not taken estrogen during the first two years of recovery. This risk decreased after three to four years of estrogen use. The women on estrogen were more likely to die in the first two years because they were at an increased risk for fatal blood clot formation. It is well established that estrogen therapy causes the blood to clot more than normal. The outcome of the HERS has influenced cardiologists to stop recommending estrogen as a therapy to prevent cardiovascular disease. The FDA and American cardiologists no longer believe that estrogen has a proven positive effect on heart disease. There is no cardiac benefit from estrogen that overshadows the risk of breast cancer.

The second study we would like to mention is the Women's Health Initiative (WHI). The Women's Health Initiative was conducted by the National Institutes of Health because of the lack of definitive evidence to support the theory that Premarin® prevented heart disease, even though doctors prescribed it for this purpose. **Dr. Jacques Rossouw, the lead project officer of the study, made this statement at the beginning of the study in 1991:**

"Long-term estrogen replacement therapy is being ardently prescribed to prevent heart disease with no evidence for these presumed benefits. Sixty-six percent (66%) of physicians who prescribe hormone replacement therapy do so at least in part to prevent coronary artery disease-an indication that is unproved and unacceptable. "

The WHI was halted after five years because of overwhelming evidence that women taking estrogen had an increased risk of heart attacks and strokes (see page 130 for more information). The HERS and Women's Health Initiative studies, both of which were controlled studies, confirmed that Premarin® does not prevent heart disease but may actually increase the risk of heart attacks in women.

The FDA and the National Institutes of Health hold the opinion that estrogen does not prevent heart disease and heart attacks in women. They also believe that it increases the risk of blood clot formation and strokes in women.

Progestins, which are added to estrogen replacement to decrease the risk of uterine cancer, have a negative effect on cholesterol. The decrease in LDL cholesterol which estrogen produces is eliminated when a progestin like Provera is added. The PEPI Study, another large, randomized, controlled study, proved this.

On the other hand, progesterone, unlike progestins, had little, if any, negative effect on LDL cholesterol. This was another finding of the PEPI Study. The PEPI Study is one of the few studies that recognized a possible difference in the effect of progestins versus progesterone. Very few studies exist that scrutinize progesterone's effect on the heart. One study explored the effect of progesterone in apes. Progestins were given to the apes, and maneuvers were utilized which were known to stimulate non-fatal heart attacks. The progestins made it easier to induce the heart changes, which led to heart attacks. The apes that were given progesterone had a different response. It was more difficult, and in some apes, virtually impossible to induce a heart attack.

Progesterone relaxes smooth muscle. Smooth muscle surrounds the walls of arteries. When smooth muscles are relaxed, blood flows smoothly through the arteries. When they are tense, it is difficult for blood to pass through. Some heart attacks are due to spasms or contractions of the arteries that supply blood to the heart. These heart attacks may be affected by progesterone and may be increased by a lack of progesterone, which could explain why heart attacks increase in women after menopause.

The graph (Fig. 1) entitled "Deaths from Heart Disease or Breast Cancer in Women in the U.S." illustrates some very interesting points. The graph correlates age in years versus percentage of deaths from heart disease and breast cancer. Breast cancer statistics are represented by the squares and the circles represent heart disease deaths. Careful evaluation of this graph reveals the following facts:

- Breast cancer does cause more deaths in women prior age 50.

- The highest rate of death from breast cancer is at age 40.

- The rate of death from breast cancer decreases after age 50.

- Heart disease deaths begin to increase at age 35.

- Deaths from heart disease are not greater than breast cancer until age 55.

Fig. 1

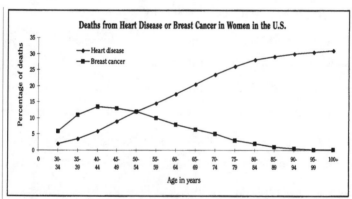

Breast cancer deaths peak between ages 40 and 50. The average age at menopause in the United States is 51, after which deaths due to coronary artery disease rise.

Source: National Center for Health Statistics: *Vital Statistics of the United States*. Vol. 11, Mortality, part B. OHHS Public Health Service Pub. No. (PHS) 90-1102, Washington, DC, US Government Printing Office, 1990.

From these facts, we can see that breast cancer is most deadly during the perimenopausal period of a woman's life. This is a time when estrogen levels are elevated and progesterone levels are low. Deaths from breast cancer decrease after menopause when estrogen levels usually decrease from the elevated perimenopausal levels. Deaths from heart disease begin to increase at age 35. Between the ages of 35 to 50 years of age, the rate of death from heart disease increases when estrogen is abundant.   What also occurs during the ages of 35 and 50 is a decline in progesterone. Could this decline in progesterone explain the increased risk of heart disease?

Finally, the graph reveals that breast cancer kills women at age 40, while heart disease kills women at age 55 and above. Women are more concerned about dying from breast cancer at age 40 than they are of dying at age 60 or 65 from heart disease. More than likely, very few women have known women who have died from a heart attack at age fifty. However, we would venture to guess that most women know someone who has died of breast cancer prior to age 55. While studies show that more women die of heart disease than breast cancer, this is only true after age 50.

What Does Prevent Heart Disease

- **Olive Oil**
- **Fish Oil**
- **Fiber**
- **Fruits and Vegetables**
- **Selenium**
- **Vitamin E**
- **Vitamin B_6 and B_{12}**
- **Folic Acid**

Points to Remember

1. Estrogen does not decrease your risk of cardiovascular disease.

2. Progesterone may have positive cardiac effects.

3. Prior to age 50, more women die of breast cancer than heart disease.

4. A decline in progesterone is associated with an increase in breast cancer and heart disease.

Chapter 11

Creating a Balance:

Balancing Estrogen and Progesterone

Debbie is a 45 year-old businesswoman. She presented complaining of hot flashes, night sweats, insomnia, fatigue, decreased libido, mood swings, thinning hair and weight gain. After a consultation with us, Debbie decided to change her diet and lifestyle. She began exercising regularly and eating organic and unprocessed food. She also began using olive oil to cook with and avoided sodas, and hormone laden dairy products and meats. Debbie incorporated soy products into her diet and started drinking a soy shake each day. Her symptoms greatly diminished and her energy level improved.

What can you do to balance your estrogen and progesterone? The choices are numerous. To help you to remember all of the choices, we have created an acronym. Just remember the word **HEALTHY.** This chapter will discuss what you can do to balance your hormones. These strategies can be used by anyone. They don't require a prescription. However, they do require that you make a decision to take control of your health.

HEALTHY

Hormonal balance

Eat whole grain, unprocessed, organic, exercise

Avoid sugar, caffeine, tobacco and alcohol

Less animal protein and stress, more plant protein, prayer and meditation

Try soy supplementation

Hormone and vitamin supplementation

You are in CONTROL

H is for Hormonal Balance

Let's take a minute and look at how our diet and lifestyle have changed over the last 200 years. The industrial revolution, which began in Europe over 200 years ago, brought about drastic changes in how food was produced, processed, stored, and distributed. These changes quickly spread to the United States.

During and following World War II, drastic changes occurred in American society. Women left home and started working in factories to build machines for the war. After the war, there were GI bills and FHA loans that allowed the returning soldiers to buy homes in cities and suburbs. The women liked being out of the home, working and pursuing educational goals.

These societal changes moved families away from family farms into cities where it was not possible to grow their own food. Markets were needed. Because men and women were busy during the week, they could not buy fresh foods everyday. They also needed foods that could be stored longer and were easier to cook. This made supermarkets necessary and the supermarkets needed food that could be easily stored and preserved for extended periods of time. Sugared breakfast cereals, snack items and instant foods are all post World War II creations. It was estimated, in 1960, that 60 % of the items in supermarkets came into existence during the 15 years following World War II.

A quote from a National Institutes of Health report sheds some light on the effects of post WWII on the American people. *"Because the changes in the dietary patterns of the more technologically developed countries, such as the United States, have been so dramatic and rapid, the people consuming these affluent diets have had little time to adapt biologically to the types and quantities of food available to them today. The longer term adverse effects of the affluent diets prevailing in these countries-- characterized by an excess of energy (calorie) dense foods rich in animal fat, partially hydrogenated vegetable oils and refined carbohydrates but lacking in whole grains, fruits and vegetables-- have become apparent only in recent decades.*

Comparisons of population groups have demonstrated a close and consistent relationship between the adoption of this affluent diet and the emergence of a range of chronic, non-infectious diseases, such as coronary heart disease, stroke, cancers, diabetes, gall stones, cavities and various bone and joint diseases."

This post World War change in American diet and lifestyle correlates with the emergence of hormone replacement therapy in women. There was no need for hormone replacement prior to World War II, because few women suffered from hormone related symptoms. Most of our grandmothers did not experience hormone-related problems. The conditions mentioned in this book are post-World War II phenomena. This gives us a clue that these conditions are not genetically related, but rather influenced by our environment, dietary habits and lifestyle. Fortunately, a woman can choose to modify most of these factors.

E is for eat whole grains, seeds and nuts.

Millet

Barley

Buckwheat

Corn

Oats

Rice

Rye

Wheat

Whole grains contain complex carbohydrates and vitamins B_1, B_2, and B_3, which are plentiful in grains. Vitamin E is found in wheat germ. The whole grain is rich in magnesium, zinc, iron, potassium, calcium, phosphorus, copper and selenium. White bread and rice do not contain the whole grain or the wheat germ. This makes them devoid of significant nutrients. The vitamins and minerals that are found naturally in whole grains are vitally important to estrogen/progesterone balance.

Vitamins E and the B vitamins are involved in the binding and elimination of estrogen by the liver. Vitamin E and B deficiencies have been associated with PMS symptoms, perimenopausal symptoms, and breast tenderness. These vitamins are also important to brain function and mood regulation. Low magnesium levels are also associated with PMS, perimenopause, menopause osteoporosis and heart disease.

Whole grains contain fiber. Fiber increases the number of carrier proteins that are available to bind and deactivate estrogen. Fiber increases the bulk and frequency of bowel movements. Estrogen is a very resilient hormone. Estrogen, which is not properly metabolized in the liver and eliminated through the bowel, is reabsorbed, and thus increases the amount of free estrogen. Several studies show that women adhering to a vegetarian diet eliminate more estrogen than non-vegetarian women. It has also been shown that high-fiber diets increase the estrogen carrier protein, which decreases free estrogen levels. A high fiber diet is associated with fewer PMS symptoms and less painful menses. The addition of a natural fiber such as Metamucil®, three times a day, may be useful until you can incorporate more fiber into your diet.

Seeds
Flax
Pumpkin
Sesame
Sunflower

These seeds are high in protein, vitamin E and essential fatty acids. They also contain fat-soluble vitamins A, D, and E, magnesium, zinc and copper. Essential fatty acids omega 3 and 9, are very important to estrogen and progesterone ratio. Omega 3 and 9 fatty acids make the cells less sensitive to estrogen. These essential fatty acids are also found in cold-water fish.

Nuts

Almonds	Hazelnuts
Brazil Nuts	Peanuts
Cashews	Pistachios
Chestnuts	Pecans
Coconuts	Walnuts
Soy	

Nuts contain proteins and fats that are essential for normal cell and hormone function. They also have small amounts of B vitamins. Nuts have high levels of vitamin E, potassium, magnesium, calcium, iron, and zinc, which are important to women's health. Because nuts are high in fat, don't eat them in abundance if you are trying to lose weight. Avoid eating nuts roasted in oil, fats, salt and other additives. Eating a handful of fresh raw nuts as a mid-morning or mid-afternoon snack is an energy-packed, protein-rich treat.

Unprocessed foods

One of our favorite books is "*What the Bible Says About Healthy Living.*" By Rex Russell. One of the principles emphasized in his book is eat food before people alter it or try to improve it. The processing of foods to make them more appealing and longer lasting has resulted in food with decreased nutritional value and has lead to an increase in diseases.

The processing of natural fats and oils into partially hydrogenated oils is detrimental to the membranes of all cells. Processed oils have been indicated in heart disease and several types of cancer, including breast cancer. These unstable fats also seem to increase the effect of estrogen on breast cells, which cause them to multiply at a greater rate.

The processing and curing of meats is also detrimental. Feeding livestock commercial feed transforms the natural fats in livestock into a more saturated and less healthy omega 6 fat. Commercial feed also decreases the amount of healthy omega 3 and 9 fats. The addition of growth hormone and estrogen to livestock feed has greatly affected women. These hormones are stored in the fat of the animals. Therefore, it is advisable to decrease your consumption of meats that are usually found in supermarkets. Animals that are allowed to roam freely, to eat grasses uncontaminated by pesticides and to be free of hormones, can be consumed safely. These meats are labeled as "free range" meats. They can be found in farmers' markets and organic food stores.

The consumption of processed commercial milk can lead to health problems. Milk and dairy products that have come from domesticated cows contain hormones. Estrogen may be used to increase the cow's weight and milk production. The milk can contain allergy-causing substances that may cause autoimmune diseases like diabetes and lupus. The pasteurization of milk kills many of the bacteria contained in milk. However, the heating involved in pasteurization destroys many enzymes needed by the body to absorb the nutrients in the milk. Milk intolerance is caused by the destruction of enzymes during the pasteurization process. Calcium is altered by the pasteurization process, and therefore cannot be efficiently absorbed by the body. Undomesticated cows consume calcium from grasses and green leafy vegetables, which are the richest source of calcium. Modern feeding methods substitute high protein, soy-based feeds for fresh green grass. Eating green vegetables gives you calcium in a form that can be properly digested and used by the body. The homogenization of milk involves crushing milk fat globules into invisible particles. Homogenization keeps milk from separating and keeps it from becoming rancid. It is believed that these small fat particles directly damage blood vessels, which in turn increases cardiovascular disease.

Fresh whole milk from cows that have grazed on non-pesticide sprayed grass do not contribute to any health problems. The butterfat in milk allows you to use the vitamins and minerals in the watery portion of the milk. The butterfat contains acids that have strong anti-carcinogenic properties, which explains why organic butter has health benefits. Butter does not increase heart disease, but margarine is associated with heart disease.

Many processed snack foods contain preservatives such as partially hydrogenated oils. These oils keep the foods from spoiling. Processed oils and fats do not become rancid like natural fats, but the body cannot metabolize them effectively. Fats or fatty acids are used to form cell membranes. These membranes decide what is allowed into cells. Abnormal cell membranes made up of processed fats may allow harmful substances into the cell, which can cause chronic diseases. Abnormal membranes may affect the way cells respond to hormones, resulting in hormonal imbalances.

Food dyes and colors may also cause adverse health effects. They can cause free radical production. Free radicals have been associated with DNA damage and the initiation of cancer. The safety of food dye and color is uncertain. Therefore, it is best to avoid them as much as possible. Eat food in its natural form. It is very hard to improve upon nature.

E Is for Eat Organic Fruits and Vegetables

Organic foods are grown in uncontaminated soil without pesticides, chemical fertilizers, or additives. These fruits and vegetables are not genetically engineered in any way. Organic fruits and vegetables that are grown in nutrient-rich soil are able to resist pests and diseases better than conventionally grown crops.

Fruits and vegetables that are conventionally grown are grown in soil that has been depleted of most of its minerals and nutrients. This makes them more susceptible to disease and pests. They require the use of pesticides and artificial fertilizer to make them flawless and visually appealing in the supermarket. The beautiful, non-organic fruits and vegetables lack the nutrients and phytochemicals (plant chemicals) that your body uses to prevent and combat disease thus increasing your risk for illness. Even though you may be eating conventional broccoli, it may not be providing you with all the nutritional benefits it should be giving you.

Whenever possible, eat organic fruits and vegetables. Non-organic foods should be washed thoroughly in soap and water before it is eaten to remove pesticides and waxes. Don't be fooled by the way organic fruits and vegetables look. Organic produce may not look as appealing as the non-organic fruits and vegetables, but they are packed with nutrients.

What fruits and vegetables should I eat?

The best answer is to eat a variety of in season, whole fruits and vegetables. More and more modern research substantiates the fact that fruits and vegetables have a wide variety of chemicals that can prevent and treat diseases and cancer. These chemicals are called phytochemicals.

Fruit is nature's perfect food. Fruits have a high water, vitamins A, C, B's and E content. Fruits contain minerals, such as calcium, magnesium, copper, manganese, and other trace minerals. Limonene, a substance found in citrus fruits, prevents cancer. Quercetin, a substance in grapes, prevents cardiovascular disease and strokes. Vitamin A or beta-carotene is an antioxidant that prevents lung cancer and possibly other cancers that are initiated by free radicals. Fruits are low in fat and high in fiber. Both of these factors are important in disease prevention.

Fruits and fruit juices may have a cooling and calming effect on the body and may be helpful in reducing body stress. Fruit consumption may help the immune system as well. Fruit juices contain natural sugars and are a good substitute for other drinks sweetened with refined sugar. Natural sugars are lower in calories. In addition, the vitamin B in fruit helps metabolize the sugar contained in fruit. Refined sugars do not contain vitamin B. Fruits are easily digested and are best eaten alone and not with other foods that take longer to pass through the digestive tract.

Vegetables - Most vegetables are high in water, essential vitamins, and minerals but low in fat and protein. Vegetables also contain carbohydrates and fiber. The fiber in vegetables allows glucose to be absorbed slowly. They do not require large amounts of insulin to be digested. Large amounts of insulin can intensify the effects of estrogen on target cells.

Many of the nutrients in vegetables may be partially lost and dissolved in the water when cooked. Eat raw vegetables or cook them as minimally as possible. Chlorophyll, which is found in most plants, is especially high in green vegetables. Magnesium is the main component of chlorophyll. Chlorophyll is produced as a result of the sun's effects on plants, and it is known to have revitalizing and refreshing effects when consumed by humans. Chlorophyll provides intestinal nourishment and helps to detoxify the liver. Because of their beta-carotene and selenium content, vegetables are thought to help reduce cancer rates.

The cruciferous family of vegetables, such as broccoli, brussel sprouts, and cauliflower, has special anti-cancer effects. These cruciferous vegetables contain 3-indole-carbinol, which facilitates estrogen metabolism. This prevents estrogen from being re-circulated into the bloodstream from the bowel.

Green leafy vegetables are probably the most nutrient-rich food found in the vegetable kingdom. They are very high in vitamins A and C and minerals like magnesium, potassium, and iron. They are also high in folic acid and calcium. Vegetables are beneficial because they provide an enormous amount of nutrition, detoxify and restore your digestive tract, support hormone function, and decrease your cancer risk with minimal caloric and fat intake.

E is for Exercise

Benefits of Exercise

Musculoskeletal system benefits

Increases muscle strength

Increases flexibility of muscles and range of joint motion

Produces stronger bones, ligaments, and tendons

Lessens chance of injury

Enhances, posture, poise and physique

Heart and blood vessel benefits

Lowers resting heart rate

Strengthens heart function

Lowers blood pressure

Improves oxygen delivery throughout the body

Increases blood supply to muscles

Enlarges the arteries to the heart

Bodily process benefits

Improves the way the body handles dietary fat

Reduces heart disease risk

Helps lower blood cholesterol and triglyceride levels

Raises levels of HDL, the "good" cholesterol

Helps improve calcium deposition in bones

Prevents osteoporosis

Improves immune function

Aids digestion and elimination

Increases endurance and energy levels

Promotes lean body mass; burns fat

Mental processes benefits

Provides a natural release from pent-up feelings

Helps reduce tension and anxiety

Improves mental outlook and self-esteem

Helps relieve moderate depression

Improves the ability to handle stress

Stimulates improved mental function

Induces relaxation and improves sleep

Increases self esteem

Longevity benefits

For every hour of exercise, there is a two-hour increase in longevity

Exercise can provide most, if not all, of the benefits that women seek from hormone replacement. Several studies show that exercise is beneficial in treating and preventing PMS, menopausal symptoms, osteoporosis, heart disease, and cancer. Other studies show that exercise is as effective as estrogen in the prevention of osteoporosis. Exercise prevents the likelihood of falls and injury from falls. Exercise decreases body fat, which decreases estrogen production. It increases blood flow to the liver and enhances detoxification of estrogen by the liver. It also increases the elimination of waste in the bowel, which in turn decreases estrogen levels. Exercise has a positive effect on mood and decreases stress, which is a concern for most women.

The benefits of exercise can be experienced with the following activities:

Gardening

Dancing

Jazzercise

Tennis

Golfing

Walking

Heavy housecleaning

Bowling

Jogging

Swimming

Weight lifting

If you want the benefits of exercise you must maintain your training heart zone for 15-20 minutes at least three times a week. To find your training zone heart rate, subtract your age from 185 beats per minute. This is your maximum heart rate. Then, take 20 from your maximum heart rate to get your minimum training zone heart rate. For example, if your age is 45, your maximum training zone heart rate would be 140 beats per minute (185-45), and your minimum training zone heart rate would be 120 beats per minute (140-20). Exercise and a healthy diet are essential if you want to get in balance hormonally, mentally, physically, and spiritually

A is for Avoid Sugar, Caffeine, Tobacco and Alcohol

Sugar that is refined from its raw state has had its vitamin B, fiber, and enzymes removed. Vitamin B is essential in the metabolism of sugar. Because refined sugars are void of vitamin B, the body must use its own supply of B vitamins. Products filled with refined sugar, which makes it difficult to consume enough vitamin B to process the sugar and carry out other functions, dominate the American diet.   This creates a vitamin B deficiency. Vitamin B is vitally important in the metabolism of estrogen. Along with metabolizing estrogen, vitamin B is important to the nervous system and helps the body cope with anxiety and stress. Sugar seems to have a profoundly negative effect on the severity of PMS symptoms. This explains why avoiding sugar and taking a B vitamin supplement alleviates or decreases PMS symptoms.

The fiber found in raw sugar assists in slowing the absorption of sugar into the bloodstream. Fiber helps the body avoid sudden elevations in blood glucose (sugar) by slowing down the absorption of sugar. Fiber also decreases the amount of time sugar remains in the intestines. This decreases the number of calories that can be absorbed from the sugar. This decrease in sugar absorption decreases the amount of insulin that is necessary to maintain proper blood glucose levels.

Sugar and refined carbohydrates increase insulin levels. Excessive insulin leads to diabetes and poor glucose control. This results in sudden shifts from elevated blood glucose levels to low glucose levels. These sudden swings can effect mood and cause aggressive behavior. Cravings are thought to be a result of alterations in blood glucose control. The high levels of insulin needed to control elevated blood glucose are detrimental when it is maintained for long periods of time. Insulin lowers the amount of estrogen carrier protein, sex hormone binding globulin (SHBG). This increases the amount of free estrogen available, which worsens any symptoms associated with excess estrogen. Excessive insulin has been associated with increased risk of cardiovascular disease.

Diabetes results when the pancreas becomes exhausted and unable to respond to elevated glucose levels. A healthy pancreas produces insulin to lower blood glucose. High-refined sugar diets place an excessive workload on the pancreas. Eventually, the pancreas can no longer produce adequate amounts of insulin and diabetes results. Women with diabetes have an increased risk of uterine and breast cancer, which is probably due to insulin's effect on free estrogen levels.

Avoid refined sugar and carbohydrates by reading labels. Almost all processed foods found in the supermarket have sugar added because it is pleasing to the taste and somewhat addictive. Fruits contain a sugar called fructose. Fructose does not increase blood sugar levels as rapidly as glucose, which is found in refined sugars. Fructose is broken down into glucose by the liver, which slows its absorption into the bloodstream. Eat foods that have been sweetened with fructose or natural raw sugar. It is questionable whether high fructose is any more nutritious than the simple sugar glucose.

Avoid simple carbohydrates that are contained in white bread, potatoes, refined pastas, and rice. These carbohydrates are rapidly broken down to glucose and raise insulin levels. Their low fiber content only intensifies the rapid rise in blood sugar. Eating whole grain breads and pastas, which contain high fiber lower insulin, levels and also provides you with the nutritional benefits of eating whole grain foods.

Caffeine - Caffeine is probably the most commonly consumed and abused drug in our society. Caffeine stimulates the central nervous system, increases blood pressure, respiration, gastrointestinal activity, stomach acid output, kidney function and mental activity. Women who have PMS should avoid caffeine. Caffeine usually worsens the anxiety and depression associated with PMS. Caffeine also can increase breast tenderness and fibrocystic breasts. Caffeine can interfere with the absorption of vitamins and minerals such as calcium and iron. Carbonated sodas are large sources of refined white sugar and caffeine. Neither have any nutritional value, and both are detrimental to hormonal balance. Sodas also contain high levels of phosphorous. Phosphorus can remove calcium from the bones, which may lead to a worsening of osteoporosis.

Alcohol - has multiple effects on hormone metabolism and can severely damage the liver if consumed in excessive amounts. The liver is responsible for the metabolizing and eliminating estrogen. As the liver's function declines, estrogen metabolism declines and estrogen levels increase. Alcoholics usually have very poor dietary habits, which creates vitamin and mineral deficiencies. Vitamins and minerals are necessary for normal hormone function. The combination of a damaged liver and vitamin and mineral deficiencies can have a devastating effect on hormonal balance. While it is true that a glass of wine a day is be beneficial, it is advisable to avoid excessive alcohol intake.

Tobacco - Women are just as susceptible to lung cancer as men. This has been demonstrated by the rise in lung cancer among women. Cigarette smoking produces free radicals. Free radicals are thought to be involved in the initiation of all types of cancers, including breast cancer. It is wise to avoid tobacco if you want to maintain your health.

L Is For Less Animal Protein and Stress

Less animal Protein - Animal protein, or meat, is a very dense form of protein that requires a lot of energy to digest. We routinely advise women to reduce or eliminate any non-organic meat from their diet. Organic meats are sometimes labeled as free range. If you are unable to eliminate milk or do not care for soymilk, we suggest organic milk and cheeses. Low fat or fat free milk and cheeses are recommended. If veggie cheese is available in your area, we recommend it. It tastes like cheese, and the kids will never know the difference.

Decreasing your consumption of meat or animal protein is not only important in decreasing your risk of estrogen associated health problems, but it is also important in decreasing heart disease and osteoporosis. Vegetarians have half the incidence of coronary artery disease as non-vegetarians. Vegetarians also have a lower incidence of hypertension, obesity, elevated cholesterol levels, arteriosclerosis, and cancers. Throughout the world, the incidence of coronary artery and heart disease correlates with a country's intake of meat.

Osteoporosis is affected by meat consumption because animal protein increases the amount of calcium excreted in the urine. Calcium is needed to neutralize the by-products of animal protein metabolism. The more meat consumed, the more calcium required. This explains why the requirement for calcium is so high in America.

Sources of plant protein include grains, beans, nuts, and green leafy vegetables. Eat a variety of unprocessed grains and vegetables. If you only eat one particular grain, legume, bean or nut, you will become deficient in one the of amino acids (protein building blocks). This explains why people in third world countries, who only eat rice or other grains in isolation, suffer from diseases caused by protein deficiency. Adding an organic egg or milk once a day, in addition to other wholesome foods, should provide a balanced diet. We are not suggesting that you must adapt a vegetarian diet to be healthy. However, eating meat three times a day is an American habit and is not a nutritional requirement.

Less stress - Stress has a direct effect on women and their hormones. Long-term stress increases free estrogen levels. Most hormone-related conditions in women are exacerbated by stress (for example, bleeding, hot flashes, cancer, etc.)

How do you eliminate or decrease stress?

1. **Identify stressors.** (see Table 1) Figure out what is causing stress in your life. In most cases, time management is the problem. Trying to live up to unrealistic societal expectations, such as being a career woman, wife, lover, mom, PTA president, chauffeur, choir member, Sunday school teacher, etc., creates stress. After you have identified your stressors you must....

2. **Eliminate or reduce the sources of stress.** Some events or situations cause stress in anyone, for example, death of a spouse or close family member. However, the effect of some stress is dependent upon your response. Some events can be devastating to one person but invigorating and exciting to another. Life is full of unexpected changes. Learn to enjoy them as you grow and mature. Also, learn to say no. Life will go on even if you don't get involved.

Table 1

Social Readjustment Rating Scale		
Rank	**Life Event**	**Mean Value**
1	Death of a spouse	100
2	Divorce	73
3	Marital separation	65
4	Jail term	63
5	Death of a close family member	63
6	Personal injury or illness	53
7	Marriage	50
8	Fired at work	47
9	Marital reconciliation	45
10	Retirement	45
11	Change in health of a family member	44
12	Pregnancy	40
13	Sex difficulties	39
14	Gain of a new family member	39
15	Business adjustment	39
16	Change in financial state	38
17	Death of a close friend	37
18	Change to different line of work	36
19	Change in number of argument with spouse	35
20	Large mortgage	31
21	Foreclosure of mortgage or loan	30
22	Change in responsibilities at work	29
23	Son or daughter leaving home	29
24	Trouble with in-laws	29
26	Wife begins or stops work	26
27	Begin or end school	26
28	Change in living conditions	25
29	Revision of personal habits	24
30	Trouble with boss	23

3. **Prayer and meditation.** Ask God for strength and wisdom. Reconnect with God and identify your purpose. Don't try to live up to the expectations of other people. God will assist you in doing what he has planned for you. Make sure you haven't excluded God from your plans. Scientific evidence shows that people that identify themselves as believing in God and prayer respond better to physical and mental stress. These people live longer than other people with similar illnesses do. People who believe in God are less likely to abuse sedatives and anti-anxiety drugs. It is good for your health to incorporate prayer and meditation in your life, if you are looking for balance and relief from stress in your life.

4. **Relaxation and breathing exercises daily.** Overwhelmed by the hustle and bustle of our society people often forget that they need rest and relaxation. There are many good books written on relaxation. One book that we recommend is *The Relaxation Response* by Herbert Benson. This book points out the benefits of focused breathing and relaxation techniques. These techniques are able to effect blood pressure, cholesterol and hormone levels. Our society has to learn how to relax and breathe if we are going to stay healthy.

5. **Enhance relationships with better communication**. Learn how to forgive. Human beings must have relationships to function happily. Infants that are not loved and held will not grow even though they are given adequate nutrition. Adults without significant relationships experience more stress and usually have poor mental and physical health. This explains why the loss of a relationship through death or divorce is rated so high as a life stressor. Sometimes, relationships are lost due to our unwillingness to forgive and communicate. It is important to maintain close relationships. Don't allow poor communication and stubbornness to destroy your relationships. Forgiveness is a gift that doesn't have to be earned. It can heal relationships, and it can also heal the person who forgives by lifting the stress of bitterness and resentment.

T is for Try Soy, Vitamin and Mineral Supplementation

Soy has received a lot of attention recently. Soybeans contain estrogen-like substances, which can attach to the estrogen receptors in cells. These substances have a very weak estrogen effect on the cells. However, with continued consumption of soy, which contains phytoestrogens and isoflavins, it can provide the positive benefits of estrogen without the negative side effects.

There are over a thousand published articles on soy. The evidence suggests:

1. Soy alleviates menopausal and perimenopausal symptoms. Symptoms such as hot flashes, night sweats, mood swings, and fatigue, vaginal dryness, and loss of libido, headaches, anxiety and insomnia may be controlled with adequate amounts of soy.

2. Soy protein may exert positive effects on bone density and reduce fractures.

3. Soy protein is safe and does not stimulate breast or uterine cells.

4. Soy may protect cells from potent estrogens, such as estradiol and xenoestrogens. Soy decreases circulating estrogen levels.

5. Soy directs the metabolism of estrogen towards inactive by-products.

6. Soy protein lowers cholesterol levels and heart disease risk (FDA approved statement October 1999)

7. Soy may decrease the risk of breast, uterine and prostate cancer by decreasing the effect of environmental estrogens and excessive amounts of estrogen made by the body.

8. Soy is a source of plant protein and fiber.

9. Soy may reduce the risk of colon cancer.

10. There may be some association with soy consumption and the reduction of Alzheimer's disease risk.

11. There is no evidence that whole soy foods increase the risk of any estrogen-sensitive cancers (FDA approved statement).

It is obvious from the aforementioned epidemiological data that soy has several important health benefits. Cancers that involve the breast, the uterus, and the prostate are dramatically lower in countries that consume significant amounts of soy. More studies are being done to critically test the benefits of soy. Over 90% of the studies confirm the association of soy with the health benefits listed above.

It is important to note that the positive benefits of soy have been associated with whole soy foods like tofu, tempeh, soybeans, soymilk, and products made from soy. Soy pills or pills that concentrate isoflavins, have not been proven to have the same positive effects of soy foods. As with most beneficial effects from foods, the whole food is required to obtain the maximum benefit.

In Asia soy is consumed along with a mineral rich fish broth. This is important because eating unfermented soy in large quantities can block the absorption of minerals. This can lead to mineral deficiencies. Vegetarians that consume tofu and bean curd as substitutes for meat may be at risk calcium, magnesium, iron, and zinc deficiencies. Fermented soy, found in tempeh and miso, do not block mineral absorption.

Most of the research shows that 60 to 80 milligrams of soy isoflavins are needed to receive significant health benefits. Asians eat approximately 160 milligrams of soy isoflavins, or one pound of tofu a day. Because it is very unlikely that most Americans will incorporate one pound of soy into the daily diet, soy shakes are an excellent way to obtain an adequate amount of isoflavins.

Vitamin and Mineral Supplementation

We believe that the best vitamin supplementation is eating whole, unprocessed, plant based foods. During the transition to a more healthy diet, vitamin supplements may be helpful in eliminating symptoms and preventing illness. We will only list the vitamins and minerals that are especially important to women. Several of the vitamins aid the liver in detoxification of environmental estrogens. They also help in metabolizing the estrogen made by the body. The result is a decrease in estrogen excess.

Vitamin B complex

Folic acid

Vitamin E

Magnesium

Vitamin D

Boron

Calcium

Manganese

Selenium

Zinc

A good way to get these vitamins and minerals in their natural form is through super foods. These are foods that have been carefully dehydrated at low temperatures to preserve their nutrients and enzymes. You may also choose to take a high potency multivitamin and a B complex vitamin each day.

H is for Hormonal Supplementation

Synthetic estrogens are not your only choice when considering hormonal replacement. Before considering hormonal replacement, first find out if you have a hormone deficiency. Saliva testing is the best method to identify what hormone you need. We do not recommend hormonal therapy unless you have had a salivary test. The next step is to replace the deficiency and monitor your progress with salivary testing.

Before discussing hormone treatment, we want to clearly state the goals of hormone therapy.

The Goals of Hormone Replacement
1. **Correct the hormone deficiency**
2. **Maintain or increase quality of life**
3. **No disruptive side effects**
4. **No increased cancer or heart disease risks**
5. **Prevention of degenerative diseases**

The following hormonal choices satisfy the goals of hormone replacement therapy.

Biest- contains **Estriol 2mg, and Estradiol .5mg.** This combination is safe and unlikely to produce side effects. It does not appear to increase breast cancer risks. It is effective in relieving hot flashes and preventing osteoporosis.

Triest- contains **Estriol 2mg, Estradiol 0.25mg. and Estrone 0.25mg.** It combines all three estrogens. This combination may be a little less desirable because estrone is thought to be associated with an increase in breast cancer risk. If this combination is used to relieve menopause symptoms, it is important to check salivary levels to make sure all three estrogens are in the normal range.

These two bio-identical estrogens (Biest and Triest) can be found in compounding pharmacies. Find a good compounding pharmacist that can answer your questions and help you find a doctor in your area.

There are also some bio-identical estrogens that are available at retail pharmacies. I recommend the use of estrogen patches that release small amounts of estrogen. These estrogens do not travel to the liver. This allows a much lower dose to be used to alleviate symptoms. The lowest amount of estrogen that can return estrogen levels back to normal is recommended.

Black Cohosh - has been used for years to alleviate menopausal symptoms. It is sold as **Remifemin**® (20 milligrams twice a day) in the U.S. and Europe. There is good evidence that black cohosh is effective in relieving hot flashes and mood disturbances. Black Cohosh is thought to bind to the estrogen receptor, however it has no estrogenic effect on female organs (the breasts and uterus). Therefore, it does not increase the risk of female cancers. One of the chemical substances in black cohosh is a precursor or building block for progesterone. It may be that black cohosh has estrogen and progesterone like effects.

Plant estrogen pills - It has been shown that soy pills containing plant estrogens do not relieve symptoms as well as soy foods and shakes. The long-term effect of taking concentrated isoflavins in a pill form is unknown. The processing and elimination of other chemicals found in the whole plant may also have detrimental effects. Some preliminary studies show that soy pills may stimulate breast tissue. Our advice is to avoid soy or plant estrogen pills until more conclusive studies on their long-term effect have been done.

Bio-identical Progesterone

Progesterone is a fat-soluble steroid hormone that can be safely used to treat a progesterone deficiency. Progesterone is best given in a micronized form. Micronized means that progesterone is contained in small microscopic packets. This form is better absorbed in the stomach and through the skin than the non-micronized form. Progesterone is FDA approved and considered to have no serious side effects. Therefore, it can be marketed and sold without a prescription in the form of a skin cream. Small amounts of progesterone are used in skin creams and cosmetics because it is a skin moisturizer.

Prometrium® is a prescription progesterone pill. This micronized progesterone pill is usually used in combination with estrogen hormone replacement. It was developed when it was determined that progestins had a negative effect on lipids produced by the liver. Progestins, like Provera®, increased the amount of bad cholesterol (LDL). Prometrium® is effective in decreasing the risk of uterine cancer in women taking estrogen. However, the other positive benefits of progesterone are not seen in women taking

Prometrium® because the liver deactivates it. The usual dose of Prometrium® is 100 to 200 milligrams, one to three times a day.

Bio-Identical Progesterone Creams

Benefits of Bio-identical Progesterone Creams

1. Easy to use
2. By-passes the stomach and the liver
3. Safe and available with or without a prescription
4. 20 to 40 milligrams once or twice a day will correct most progesterone deficiencies
5. Can be used from puberty through menopause
6. Compounded progesterone creams prescribed by a doctor, can vary the amount of progesterone as needed.

Because progesterone creams are not regulated, make sure that the cream:

1. Contains U.S. Pharmaceutical grade progesterone
2. Contains at least 400 milligrams of progesterone per ounce and no more than 500 milligrams per ounce
3. Does not contain wild yam only
4. Is laboratory tested to confirm the progesterone content

Progesterone creams are very popular with women. They are popular because they provide amazing relief from symptoms associated with hormonal imbalances. Very few physicians are aware of the therapeutic benefits of progesterone. Many physicians are confused by the publicized benefits of progesterone because progestins do not have the same benefits.

Table 2 illustrates the tremendous differences between bio-identical progesterone and synthetic progestins. Progestins are compounds found in birth control pills, Prempro® and Provera®. Understanding the differences is essential to understanding how bio-identical progesterone can be beneficial to women.

Comparison of Bio-identical Progesterone vs. Progestins

Table 2	Bio-Identical Progesterone	Progestins
Increases sodium and water in cells		X
Causes loss of minerals and electrolytes from cells		X
Causes depression		X
Causes facial hair and loss of scalp hair		X
Elevate blood sugar		X
Cause allergic reactions		X
Causes acne and skin rashes		X
Increases birth defect risks		X
Increases risk of blood clots		X
Protects against endometrial cancer	X	X
Protects against breast cancer	X	
Normalizes sex drive	X	

Condition	Bio-identical Progesterone	Progestin
Causes less facial hair growth	X	
Regrowth of scalp hair	X	
Improves lipid levels	X	
Improves in vitro fertilization	X	
Assists in new bone formation	X	Some
Decrease risk of coronary artery spasm	X	
Increases action of thyroid hormone	X	
Prevents implantation of fertilized egg		X
Is essential for successful pregnancy	X	
Is essential for normal nerve function	X	
Restores normal sleep patterns	X	
Building block for other hormones	X	
Relieves hot flashes	X	slightly

Adapted from *What Your Doctor May not Tell You About Perimenopause,* by, J. Lee

If you are interested in taking bio-identical progesterone, it is important to:

1. Find a doctor who is knowledgeable and comfortable with using bio-identical or natural progesterone.

2. If your doctor is interested in learning about the use of bio-identical progesterone give him/her a copy of this book. There are medical references at the end of this book that may be helpful to your doctor.

3. Get a baseline saliva test to confirm whether you have estrogen excess or a progesterone deficiency.

4. Use a progesterone cream prescribed by your physician that can be formulated at a compounding pharmacy.

5. Use an over the counter progesterone cream that meets the requirements listed previously.

6. Use the recommended dose during the recommended time of the menstrual cycle.

7. Avoid overdosing because you can create symptoms of progesterone deficiency.

8. Retest saliva hormone levels every 6-12 months to monitor replacement therapy and prevent overdosing.

The fat under the skin absorbs approximately 10% of the amount of progesterone applied to the skin. This is ten times the amount absorbed as compared to progesterone pills. The body produces 2 to 4 milligrams of progesterone a day. Applying 20 to 40 milligrams a day will replace what the body normally makes. If a cream contains 400 to 450 milligrams of progesterone an ounce, 1/4 to 1/2 of a teaspoon in two divided doses will provide an appropriate amount of progesterone. Some women will need to apply more to control their symptoms initially.   After several months of use, it is advisable to decrease the dose of progesterone. Progesterone does not have any adverse side effects. However, after several months, progesterone collects in the fat tissue. This can lead to an abnormally high level of progesterone. When progesterone reaches an extremely elevated level, the body no longer responds to the progesterone. As a result, the progesterone may be converted to estrogen in attempt to achieve balance. This of course makes the estrogen excess worse. Typically, women will notice the return of their symptoms. The level can be returned to normal by discontinuing the progesterone cream for two to three months.

How to Use Bio-Identical Progesterone Cream

The GOAL of progesterone replacement is to re-establish the NORMAL estrogen/progesterone ratio.

1. Begin using progesterone on the 12th day after the start of the previous menstrual cycle.

   Progesterone production normally occurs around day 12 to 14 of the menstrual cycle.

2. Continue to use the progesterone until day 26 of the menstrual cycle.

3. The menstrual cycle should begin a few days after discontinuing the progesterone.

4. If your menstrual cycle starts prior to day 26, stop using the progesterone. Count the day of menstrual flow as day 1 and begin the progesterone cream again on day 12 to 14. With continued use, the menstrual cycle should lengthen and extend beyond 26 days.

5. Depending upon the severity of symptoms and the deficiency detected with saliva testing, use between ¼ to ½ of a teaspoon of progesterone twice a day. This equates to 20 to 40 milligrams per dose.

6. Apply the cream to areas on the body that have thin skin and many blood vessels. This includes the hands and feet, the neck, the inner arms, the inner thighs and the breast. Rotate sites to avoid saturating one area. (Example: Hands in the morning, and neck in the evening.)

7. Applying $1/8^{th}$ to $¼^{th}$ of a teaspoon directly on the abdomen when you are experiencing menstrual cramps relieves the cramps in less than 20 minutes in most women. In general, menstrual cramps will improve with the use of progesterone.

Progesterone use in Menopause

1. Use ¼ to ½ of a teaspoon twice a day for three weeks each month. During the fourth week, do not use progesterone. If your symptoms are intolerable during the fourth week you may use half of your usual dose. It is important to take a break from the progesterone to avoid saturating its receptors. If the body becomes saturated, the progesterone will be ineffective in relieving symptoms.

2. After approximately three months of using bio-identical progesterone, most women can cut their usual dose by one half and not experience significant symptoms.

3. If you want to stop taking estrogen, inform your healthcare provider. You should taper your dose gradually. Remember your body has been accustomed to high levels of estrogen. While using the progesterone as recommended, taper the estrogen dose by:

   - Taking your usual dose of estrogen every other day for one to two months.

   - If there are no significant symptoms, begin taking the estrogen every third day for one to two months.

- Next, take the estrogen every fourth day for one to two months.
- By the end of three to six months, you should not require estrogen.

During the tapering, it is also recommended that you incorporate the other changes mentioned in this chapter. The addition of soy foods and soy shakes will be especially helpful in preventing the return of hot flashes.

Progesterone can be used to prevent or treat several conditions that may be influenced by a progesterone deficiency or an excess of estrogen. It is extremely important that you do not attempt to diagnose and treat yourself. You must see your doctor or health care provider once a year to receive a proper screening for illnesses. We strongly suggest that you find a healthcare provider that will assist you in balancing your hormones using some of the recommendations in this book.

Progesterone may be used in the following conditions:

PMS - Use the cream starting on day 12. Day 12 is twelve days after your last period began. You may need to use it only once a day two weeks prior to your period and two to three times a day during the week prior to your period. Progesterone often relieves the headaches that occur prior to the menstrual cycle. It is important to make sure that your symptoms do not meet the criteria for depression or any other psychiatric illness. If the symptoms are constant and not related to the two weeks prior to your menses another diagnosis must be considered.

Perimenopause - Progesterone is useful in treating, most, if not all the symptoms associated with the perimenopausal period. However, sometimes other methods are needed to properly treat these symptoms. Women with excessive bleeding may need Provera® or Depo-Provera® to stop the bleeding. Progesterone may be helpful after the heavy bleeding is under control. Sometimes an endometrial ablation, an outpatient surgical procedure that involves the destruction of the uterine lining by applying heat or cold, may be needed to control bleeding. In a small percentage of women, a hysterectomy may have to be done to control severe, heavy vaginal bleeding. However, this is needed in a very small number of women.

During perimenopause it is important to report to your doctor any persistent abdominal pain or pressure, abnormal bleeding or breast lumps. Bio-identical progesterone is useful in prevention and early treatment of many perimenopausal conditions. The sooner you are diagnosed, the more likely progesterone will be able to control and prevent the progression of symptoms which might lead to more invasive treatments.

Breast pain and fibrocystic breast - Bio-identical progesterone has been shown to alleviate breast pain in 96% of women. In mild to moderate fibrocystic breasts, bio-identical progesterone reverses the condition in 85% of women.

Infertility - Progesterone is vitally important in the maintenance of an early pregnancy. Adding progesterone can be beneficial in supporting an early pregnancy in women with progesterone deficiencies.

Fibroids - Fibroids that are small (4 centimeters or less) can be prevented from growing and actually made smaller by using progesterone.

Endometriosis - Mild endometriosis can be treated with bio-identical progesterone. It is effective in controlling the pain and bleeding associated with endometriosis.

Menopause - The symptoms of menopause that are due to a relative progesterone deficiency can be treated with bio-identical progesterone. Saliva testing can identify elevated estrogen levels. Using progesterone is effective in alleviating hot flashes and other menopausal symptoms in 83% of postmenopausal women. Progesterone restores the normal estrogen/progesterone ratio that is disrupted by elevated levels of estrogens in menopausal women.

Osteoporosis - Some studies have shown that bio-identical progesterone plays a role in building and maintaining bone. This has not been well studied. Logically, it would make sense that bone would benefit from hormonal balance.

Other Supplements

Chasteberries (Vitex) - stimulates the pituitary gland to produce a hormone called leutenizing hormone, which in turn stimulates the production of progesterone. Vitex has been safely used for years in the treatment of many of the conditions mentioned above. Chasteberries have been labeled the great female regulator. One studied showed that 175 milligrams of Chasteberry was as effective as vitamin B_6 in relieving PMS symptoms.

DHEA

Dehydroepiandrosterone (DHEA) - is a steroid made in the adrenal glands. Salivary testing often shows a decreased level in perimenopausal and postmenopausal women. This hormone is primarily converted to androgens in males but it is present in significant amounts in women. The effect of DHEA has not been well studied in women. DHEA is believed to be involved in the maintenance of bone density. It also increases immune function, energy levels, the feeling of well-being and sex drive. It may be advisable to supplement women low in DHEA with 5 to 10 milligrams of DHEA a day. It is important to monitor DHEA levels. Elevated levels can lead to acne, hair loss and growth of facial hair.

Y is for YOU ARE IN CONTROL

We would like to close by sharing the following story. There once was a lead caterpillar named Harry. The other caterpillars instinctively followed him. He was good at helping the other caterpillars find food. One day, a little boy placed the lead caterpillar and the others on top of a jar. Inside the jar was an ample amount of food.

The lead caterpillar confused and frightened began to go in circles on top of the jar. The other caterpillars continued to follow him even though they were starving. Eventually, all the caterpillars died from starvation despite the fact that there was food inside the jar. In closing, DON'T BE A CATERPILLAR! Trust your intuition. Take control of your life and make informed decisions about your health.

About The Authors

Eldred B. Taylor M.D., originally from Nashville, Tennessee, received his Bachelor of Science degree from Vanderbilt University in Nashville, Tennessee. He earned his M.D. from Emory University School of Medicine. He also completed his internship and residency specialty training in obstetrics and gynecology at Emory in 1990. He is also Assistant Clinical Professor at Emory University School of Medicine.

Today, Dr. Taylor practices women's healthcare with special attention to caring for body, mind and soul of the patient. Dr. Taylor combines his exceptional training in conventional obstetrics and gynecology and his experience with alternative therapies, to provide comprehensive patient focused care. He believes that patients and doctors should work together in partnership to achieve the best possible treatment outcome. Dietary and lifestyle changes along with safe, effective natural therapies can solve many problems, avoiding the need for surgery and synthetic medication, which can produce side effects. However, when surgery and medications are needed, Dr. Taylor uses diet, lifestyle changes, and natural therapies to enhance their benefits.

Dr. Taylor and his wife Ava Bell-Taylor, M.D., a board certified psychiatrist, publish a newsletter, Natural Woman, four times each year. Natural Woman covers all aspects of women's health including body, mind and soul. He and his wife are the coauthors of the book, *Are Your Hormones Making You Sick*. Dr. Eldred Taylor is a very well known speaker. He is frequently invited to speak to medical, church, and civic organizations.

Dr. Ava Bell-Taylor, M.D. has practiced psychiatry for the past ten years. She received her B.S. degree from Spelman College. She later received her M.D. from Morehouse School of Medicine. Dr. Bell-Taylor completed an internship in family practice at Floyd Medical Center. She also completed a residency in psychiatry at Emory University. Dr. Taylor specializes in mind/body medicine, which places special emphasis on how the mind contributes to medical illnesses. She is the founder of Physicians Natural Medicine Institute, Inc., which is a resource center for doctors and patients who desire information regarding integrative medicine.

The Taylors reside in Stone Mountain, Georgia with their two children, Winston and Ava Patrice.

Bibliography

1. Speroff L, Glass R, Kase N. *Clinical Gynecologic Endocrinology and Infertility.* Baltimore:Williams &Wilkins,1994

2. Bardin CW, Milgrom E, Mauvais-Jarvis. *Progesterone and Progestins.* New York:Reven Press, 1983

3. Mishell D, Davajan V. *Infertility, Contraception & Reproductive Endocrinology.*Oradell, New Jersey:Medical Economics Books, 1986

4. Wright J, Morgenthaler J. *Natural Hormone Replacement.* Petaluma:Smart Publications, 1997

5. Love S., Lindsey K. *Dr. Susan Love's Hormone Book.* New York:Random House., 1997

6. Lee J. *What Your Doctor May Not Tell You About Premenopause.* New York:Warner Books, 1999

7. Lee J. *What Your Doctor May Not Tell You About Menopause.* New York:Warner Books, 1996

8. Murray M, Pizzorno J. *Encyclopedia of Natural Medicine.* California:Prima Publishing, 1998

9. Northrup C. *Women's Bodies, Women's Wisdom.* New York:Bantam Books, 1998

10. Murray M. *Encyclopedia of Nutritional Supplements.* California:Prima Publishing, 1996

11. Russell R. *What the Bible Says About Health Living*. California: Regal Publishing, 1996

12. Duke J. *The Green Pharmacy*. New York: St. Martin's Press, 1997

13. Barnard N. *Food for Life: How the New Four Food Groups Can Save Your Life*. New York:Three Rivers Press, 1993

14. Simone C. *Cancer and Nurtition*. New York: Avery Publishing Group Inc., 1994

15. Haas E. *Staying Healthy with Nutrition*. The Complete Guide to Diet & Nutritional Medicine. California: Celestial Arts Publishing, 1992

16. Cabot W., Germano C. *The Osteoporosis Solution*. New York: Kensington Publishing Corp., 1996

17. Erasmus U. *Fats that Heal Fats that Kill*. BC Canada:Alive Books. 1999

18. Weil A. *Natural Health, Natural Medicine*. New York: Houghton Mifflin Company, 1998

19. Pert C. *Molecules of Emotion*. New York: Scribner, 1997

20. Chopra D. Ageless Body, Timeless Mind. New York: Three Rivers Press, 1993

21. Noteloveitz m. Osteoporosis: Prevention, Diagnosis and Management. PCI, 1997

References

Estrogen, Progesterone and Hormonal Imbalance

1. Bardin CW, Milgrom E, Mauvais-Jarvis. *Progesterone and Progestins.* New York:Reven Press, 1983
2. Lobo R, Fraser I. Update on Progestin Therapy. Consensus Development Conference sponsored by College of Physicians and Surgeons of Columbia University. *Journal of Reproductive Medicine.* 1999:44(2) supplement
3. Maxson W, Hargrove J. Bioavailability of oral micronized progesterone. *Fertil Steril* 1985;44:622
4. Barensten R , Weijer V. Progestogens:pharmacological characteristics and clinically relevant differences. *Eur Menopause J* 3(4)266-272, 1996
5. Martorano J, Ahlgrimm M. Differentiating between natural progesterone and synthetic progestogens:clinical implications for premenstrual syndrome and perimenopause management. *Comp Ther.* 1998;24(6/7):336-339
6. Sauer M. Progesterone therapy: modern uses and treatment alternatives. *Contemporary Ob/Gyn.* 1998;Aug. supplement
7. Bourgain C, Devroey P. Effects of natural progesterone on the morphology of endometrium in patients with primary ovarian failure. *Human Reproduction.* 1990;5(5);537-543
8. Archer D. Progesterone: Pharmacokinetics and physiologic effects on the central nervous system. *Contemporary Ob/Gyn*1998;September,Supplement

9. Murray J. Natural progesterone:What role in women's health care? *Women Health Primary Care.*1998; 1(8):671-678

10. Stanczyk F. Pharmacokinetics of progesterone administered by the oral and parenteral routes. *J Reprod Med* 1999;44:141-147

11. Lobo R. Progestogen metabolism. *J Reprod Med 1999;44:148-152*

12. *Bouchard P.* Progesterone and the progesterone receptor. *J Reprod Med* 1999;44:153-157

13. Speroff L. Role of progesterone in normal breast physiology. *J Reprod Med* 1999;44:172-179

14. Zava D. Estrogen and progestin bioactivity of foods, herbs, and spices.*P.S.E.B.M.* 1998;217:368-377

15. Kant A, Schatzkin A, A prospective study of diet quality and mortality in women. *JAMA* 2000;283(16):2109-2115

16. Armstrong B, Brown J Diet and reproductive hormones: a study of vegetarian and non-vegetarian postmenopausal women. *JNCI* 1981; 67:761-767

17. Rose D, Boyer A. Effect of a low-fat diet on hormone levels in women with cystic breast disease. Serum steroid and gonadotropins. *JNCI* 1987; 78:623-626

18. Goldin B, Aldercreutz H, Estrogen excretion patterns and plasma levels in vegetarian and omnivorous women. *N. Engl J Med* 1982; 307: 1542-1547

19. Barnard N, Scialli A. Diet and sex-hormone binding globulin, dysmenorrhea, and premenstrual syndrome. *Obstet Gynecol* 2000;95:245-50

20. Aldercreutz H. Western diet and western diseases:some hormonal and biochemical mechanisms and associations. *Scan J Clin Lab Invest* 1990; 50 Suppl 201:3-23

Salivary Testing

22. Groeneveld FP, Bareman FP. Determinants of first prescription of hormone replacement therapy. A follow-up study among 1689 women aged 45-60 years. *Maturitas* 1994 Dec: 20(2-3):81- 9

23. Plymate SR, Moore DE. Sex hormone-binding globulin changes during the menstrual cycle. *J Clin Endocriol Metabolism* 1985 Nov;61(5):993-6

24. Adlercreutz H. Western diet and western diseases: some hormonal and biochemical mechanisms and associations. *Scand J Lab Invest.* 1990;50, Suppl 201:3-23

25. Moumib N, Sultan C, et. al Correlation between free plasma estradiol and estrogens determined by bioluminescence in saliva, plasma, and urine during spontaneous and FSH stimulated cycles in women. *J Steroid Biochem* 1988 Nov;31(5):861-5

26. Shannon IL, Prigmore JR. The 17-hydroxycorticosteroids of parotid fluid, serum and urine, following intramuscular injection of repository corticotrophin. *J Clin Endocrinol* 1959; 19:1477-80

27. Vining R, McGinley R. Hormones in saliva: Mode of entry and consequent implications for clinical interpretation.*Clin. Chem* 1983;29(10):1752-1756

28. Vining R, McGinley R. The measurement of hormones in saliva: possibilities and pitfalls. *J Steroid Biochem.*1987;27(1-3):81-94

29. Raid-Fahmy D, Read G. Salivary steroid assays for assessing variation in endocrine activity.*J. Steroid Biochem.*1983;19(1):265-272

30. Ellison P. Measurement of salivary progesterone.*Annals New York academy of Sciences*

31. Raid -Fahmy D, Read GF. Determination of ovarian steroid hormone levels in saliva. An overview. *J Reproduct Med* 1987;32: 254-72

32. Darne J, McGarrigle H. Saliva oestradiol, oestrone and progesterone levels in pregnancy:spontaneous labour at term preceded by a rise in the saliva oestriol: progesterone ratio. *British Journal of Obstetrics and Gynaecology.*1987;94:227-235

33. Mandel ID.The diagnostic uses of saliva. *J Oral Pathol Med* 1990;19:119-225

34. Wingfield M. O'Herlihy C. Follicular and luteal phase salivary progesterone profiles in women with endometriosis and infertility. *Gyne Endo* 8(1):21-5, 1994 Mar

35. Finn MM, Gosling JP. The frequency of salivary progesterone sampling and the diagnosis of luteal phase insufficiency. *Gyne Endo* 6(2): 127-34, 1992 Jun

36. Tallon DF, Gosling JP. Direct solid phase enzyme immunoassay of progesterone in saliva. *Clin Chem* 30(9):1507-1, 1984 Sep

37. Smith RG, Paige KB. Saliva as a matrix for measuring free androgens: Comparison with serum androgens in polycystic ovarian disease. *Fertil Steril* 31:513;1979

38. Zorn JR, McDonough PG. Salivary progesterone as an index of the luteal function. *Fertil Steril* 41:248, 1984

39. Raid-Fahmy D. Salivary progesterone for investigating ovarian activity. *Front. Oral Physiol* (5):110-123 (Karger, Basel 1984)

40. Luisi M, Franchi F. Salivary steroid measurement: an alternative approach to plasma assays in assessing endocrine function. *Front. Oral Physiol.* (5):124-154;(Karger, Basel 1984)

41. Luisi M, Franchi F. Radioimmunoasay for progesterone in human saliva During the menstrual cycle. *Journal of Steroid Biochemistry* (14):1069-1073;1981

42. Donaldson A, Jeffcoate SB. Assays of oestradiol and progesterone in saliva in the assessment of ovarian function. *Front. Oral Physiol.*.(5):80-86: (Karger, Basel 1984)

43. Choe JK, Kahn-Daewood FS. Progesterone and estradiol in the saliva and plasma during the menstrual cycle. Am. J. Obstet. Gynecol. 147:557, 1983

44. Lu Y, Bently GR. Salivary estradiol and progesterone levels in conception and nonconception cycles in women:evaluation of a new assay for salivary estradiol. *Fertil Steril* 1999 May; 71(5):863-8

45. Worthman CM, Stallings JF. Sensitive salivary estradiol assay for monitoring ovarian function. *Clin Chem* 1990 Oct;36(10): 1769-73

46. Banerjee S. Levitz M, Rosenberg CR. On the stability of salivary progesterone under various conditions of storage. *Steroids* 1985 Dec;46(6):967-74

47. Vuorento T, Lahti A. Daily measurements of salivary progesterone reveal a high rate of anovulation in healthy students. *Scand J Clin Lab Invest* 1989 June;49(4);395-401

48. Ellison P, Lipson S. Salivary estradiol-a viable alternative? (letter) Fertil Steril 1999; 72(5):951-2 Nov

PMS, Fibroids, Breast Pain, Endometriosis, and Perimenopause

49. Schmidt P, Nieman L. Differential behavioral effects of gonadal steroids in women with and in those without premenstrual tension. *N Engl J Med* 1998;338:209-16

50. Rapkin A, Morgan M. Progesterone metabolite allopregnanolone in women with premenstrual syndrome. *Obstet Gynecol* 1997;709-14

51. Mortola J. From GnRH to SSRI's and beyond: weighing the options for drug therapy in premenstrual syndrome. *Medscape Women's Health* 2(10), 1997

52. Pray S. PMS: a disorder that is diagnosable. *U.S. Pharmacist* 23 (9):1998

53. Maxson W. The use of progesterone in the treatment of PMS. *Clinical Obstetrics and Gynecology*, Vol. 30, No. 2:June 1987

54. Baker E, Best R. Efficacy of progesterone vaginal suppositories in alleviation of nervous symptoms in patients with premenstrual syndrome. *Journal of Assisted reproduction and Genetics* 1995; (12) 3:205-09

55. Singh B, Berman B. Incidence of premenstrual syndrome and remedy usage: a national probability sample study. *Altern Ther Health Med.* 1998;4(3);75-79

56. Bicikova' M, Hill M. Allopregnanolone in women with premenstrual syndrome. *Horm. Metab. Res.* 30 (1998)227-230

57. Buderi D, Wan L. Is evening primrose oil of value in the treatment of premenstrual syndrome? *Controlled Clin Trials* 1996;17:60-68

58. Freeman EW, Rickels K. A double-blind trial of oral progesterone, alprazolam, and placebo in treatment of severe premenstrual syndrome. *JAMA.* 1995;274:51-57

59. Seippel L, Backstrom T. Luteal-phase estradiol relates to symptom severity in patients with premenstrual syndrome. *J Clin Endocrinol Metab* 83: 1988-1992, 1998

60. Dunnerstein L,Spencer-Gardner C, Progesterone and the premenstrual syndrome: a double blind crossover trial. *Br Med J* 1998; 290:1617-23

61. Freeman E.Premenstrual syndrome:current perspectives on treatment and etiology. *Current opinions in Obstetrics and Gynecology* 1997, 9:147-153

62. Pearlstein T. Hormones and depression: what are the facts about premenstrual syndrome, menopause, and hormone replacement therapy. *Am J Obstet Gynecol* 1995;173:646-53

63. Freeman E, Rickels K. Ineffectiveness of progesterone suppository treatment of premenstrual syndrome. *JAMA.* 1990;264:349-53

64. Dalton K, The aetiology of premenstrual syndrome is with the progesterone receptors. *Medical Hypothesis* (1990) 31, 323-327

65. Debold J, Frye C. Progesterone and the neural mechanisms of hamster sexual behavior. *Psychoneuroendocrinology*, Vol. 19 Nos. 5-7, pp 563-579 1994

66. Rubinow D, Hoban C. Changes in plasma hormones across the menstrual cycle in patients with menstrually related mood disorder and in control subjects. *Am J Obstet Gynecol* 1988;158;5-11

67. Herzog A. Intermittent progesterone therapy and frequency of complex partial seizures in women with menstrual disorders. *Neurology* 1986;36:1607-1610

68. Backstro T, Carstensen H. Estrogen and progesterone in plasma in relation to premenstrual tension. *Journal of Steroid Biochemistry.*1974;5:257-260

69. Ling F, Mortola J. Premenstrual syndrome and premenstrual dysphoric disorder;scope, diagnosis, and treatment. *Association of Professors of Gynecology and Obstetrics* 1998;October

70. Majewska M,Harrison N. Steroid hormone metabolites are barbituate-like modulators of the GABA receptor. *Science* 1986;232:1004-7

71. Backstrom, T, Carnestensen H. FSH,LH, TeBG capacity, estrogen and progesterone in women with premenstrual tension during the luteal phase. *J Steroid Biochem.* 7: 473-476.
72. Chiaffarino F, Parazzini Fabio. Diet and uterine myomas. *Obstet Gynecol* 1994;94:395-8
73. Sitruck-Ware R, *Treatment of benign breast diseases by progesterone applied topically.*
74. Alderman E. Breast problems in the adolescent. *Conemporary Ob/Gyn* May1999; 57-74
75. Berga S. et. Al. Managing the perimenopause: the new understanding and its clinical application. *Cont Ob/Gyn.*1999;(supplement)Sept.

Menopause

76. Hargrove JT, Osteen K. An alternative method of hormone replacement therapy using natural sex steroids. *Infertility and Reproductive Medicine Clinics of North America.* 1995;6(4):653-673
77. Newton K, Lacroix A. The physician's role in women's decision making about hormone replacement therapy. *Obstet Gynecol* 1998;92:580-4
78. Col N, Legato M. HRT:new data, continuing controversies. *Patient Care.* 1998; December:92-94
79. Taylor M. Alternatives to conventional HRT: phytoestrogens and botanicals. *Contemporary Ob/Gyn.*1999;June: 27-50
80. Leonetti H, Anasti N. Natural progesterone cream for vasomotor symptoms and postmenopausal bone loss. *Obstet Gynecol* 1999;94:225-8

81. Paganini-Hill A, Henderson V. Estrogen replacement therapy and risk of alzheimer disease. *Arch Intern Med.*1996;156:2213-2217

82. Jones K. Menopause and cognitive function: estrogens and alternative therapies. *Clinical Obstetrics and Gynecology.* 2000;43(1):198-206

83. Groeneveld FP, Bareman FP. Determinants of first prescription of hormone replacement therapy. A follow-up study among 1689 women aged 45-60 years. *Maturitas* 1994;20 (2-3):81-9

84. Oddens BJ, Boulet MJ. Hormone replacement therapy among Danish women aged 45-65 years: prevalence, determinants, and compliance. *Obstet Gynecol* 1997;90(2):269-77

85. Jones KP. Menopause: new management options. *Clinical Obstetrics and Gynecology* 2000; 43(1):156-183

Estrogen, Progesterone and Cancer

86. Pujol P, Hilsenbeck S. Rising levels of estrogen receptor in breast cancer over 2 decades. *Cancer* 1994; 74:1601-6

87. Clark GM, McGuire W. Progesterone receptors and human breast cancer. *Breast Cancer Research and Treatment.* 1983;3:157-163

88. Cowan L, Gordis L. Breast cancer incidence in women with a history of progesterone deficiency. *American Journal of Epidemiology.* 1981;114(2):209-217

89. Bu S, Yin D. Progesterone induces apoptosis and up-regulation of p53 expression in human ovarian carcinoma cell lines. *Cancer* 1997;79:1944-50

90. Kandouz M, Siromachkova M. Antagonism between estradiol and progestin on BCL-2 expression in breast cancer cells. *Int. J. Cancer.* 1996;68:120-125

91. Zava D, Blen M. Estrogenic activity of natural and synthetic estrogens in human breast cancer cells in culture. *Environ Health Perspect* 1997;105(Suppl 3):637-645

92. Mohr P, Wang D. Serum progesterone and prognosis in operable breast cancer. *British Journal of Cancer.* 1996;73:1552-1555

93. Calle E. Breast cancer and HRT:a careful look at the epidemiologic evidence. *Women's Health Primary Care* 1999;2(5 suppl 1):7-14

94. Boman K, Strang P. The influence of progesterone and androgens on the growth of endometrial carcinoma. *Cancer* 1993;71:3565-9

95. Persson I. Cancer risk in women receiving estrogen-progestin replacement therapy. *Maturitas* 1996;23(Suppl):S37-45

96. Goldstein F, Stampfer M. Postmenopausal hormone therapy and mortality. *N Engl J Med.* 1997;336(25):1769-75

97. Rodriguez C, Calle E. Estrogen replacement therapy and fatal ovarian cancer. *Am J Epidemiol.* 1995;141(9):828-35

98. Cobleigh M. Norlock F. Hormone replacement therapy and high S phase in breast cancer. *JAMA* 1999;281:1528-1530

99. Garg P Kerlikowske K. Hormone replacement therapy and the risk of epithelial ovarian carcinoma: a meta-analysis. *Obstet Gynecol* 1998;92:472-9

100. Formby B, Wiley T. Progesterone inhibits growth and induces apoptosis in breast cancer cells: inverse effects on Bcl-2 and p53. *Annals of Clinical and Laboratory Science.* 1998;28(6):360-8

101. Goldstein S. Breast cancer prevention, an evaluation of methods. *Ob Management.* 2000 (July) 72-86

102. Lichtenstein P, Holm N. Environmental and heritable factors in the causation of cancer--analysis of cohorts of twins from Sweden, Denmark, and Finland. *N Engl J Med* 2000:343:78-85

103. Guzman RC, Rajkumar L. Hormonal prevention of breast cancer::mimicking the protective effect of pregnancy. *Proc Natl Acad Sci USA* 1999;96(5):2520-5

104. Gajdos C, Tartter P. Breast cancer diagnosed during hormone replacement therapy. *Obstet Gynecol* 2000;95:513-8

Osteoporosis

105. Prior JC. Progesterone as a bone-trophic hormone. *Endocrine Reviews.* 1990; 11(2):386-398

106. Hudson T. Osteoporosis:an overview for clinical practice. *Research Reviews.*Journal of Naturopathic Medicine. 7(1)

107. Prior JC. Progesterone and the prevention of osteoporosis. *The Canadian J of Ob/Gyn and Women's Health Care.*1991;3(4):178-184

108. Abdalla HI, Hart DM. Prevention of bone mineral loss in postmenopausal women by norethindrone. Obstet Gynecol 1985;666:789-92

109. Panay N, Studd John. Do progestogens and progesterone reduce bone loss? *Menopause:The Journal of the North American Menopause Society.* 1996;3(1):13-19

110. Prior JC, et al. Spinal bone loss and ovulatory disturbances. *New Engl J Med* 1990;323:1221-7

111. Kaunitz AM. Long-acting hormonal contraception: assessing impact on bone density, weight, and mood. *Int J Fertil Womens Med.*1999;44(2):110-7

112. Meunier PJ. Evidence-based medicine and osteoporosis: a comparison of fracture risk reduction data from osteoporosis randomized clinical trials. *Int L Clin Prac* 1999 Mar;53(2):122-99

113. Lloyd T, Hershey M. Penn State Young Women's Health Study. *Pediatrics* 2000;106:40-44

114. Seeley JA, Browner WS. Estrogen replacement therapy and mortality among older women. The study of osteoporotic fractures. *Arch Intern Med* 1997;157(19):2181-7

115. Lindsay R. Scietific clinical developments in osteoporosis. *Medscape Women's Health* 1999; 4(6)

116. New S. Nutritional factors influencing the development and maintenance of bone health throughout the life cycle. *World Congress on Osteoporosis* 2000

117. Burghardt M. Exercise at menopause: critical difference. *Medscape Women's Health* 1999; 4(1)

118. Wyshak G, Frisch RE. Carbonated beverages, dietary calcium, the dietary calcium/phosphorus ratio, and bone fractures in girls and boys. *J Adolese Health* 1994;15(3);210-5

119. Feskanich D, Willett WC. Milk, dietary calcium, and bone fracture in women: a 12-year prospective study. *Am J Public Health* 1997;876):992-7

120. Gray K. Estrogens, progestins, and bone *World Congress on Osteoporosis 2000*

Phytoestrogens

121. King L, Carr B. Phytoestrogens: fact or fiction. Contemporary Ob/Gyn. 1998(Sept):49-60

122. Albertazzi P, Bonaccorsi G. The effect of dietary soy supplementation an hot flushes. Obstet Gynecol 1998;91(1):6-11

123. Washburne S, Burke G. Effect of soy protein supplementation on serum lipoproteins, blood pressure,

and menopausal symptoms in perimenopausal women. Menopause 1999 Spring; 6(1):7-13

124.   Tham D, Gardner C. Clinical review 97: potential health benefits of dietary phytoestrogens: a review of the clinical, epidemiological, and mechanistic evidence. *J Clin Endocrin and Met* 1998 Jul;83(7):2223-35

125.   Knight D, Eden J. A review of the clinical effects of phytoestrogens. *Obstet Gynecol.* 1996 May: 87(5 Pt 2): 897-904

126.   Ingram D, Sanders K. Case control study of phyto-oestrogens and breast cancer. *Lancet* 1997 Oct 4; 350(9083):904-4

127.   Zheng W., Custer D. Urinary excretion of isoflavonoids and the risk of breast cancer. *Cancer Epidemiology Biomarkers Prev* 1999 Jan;8(1):35-40

128.   Stephens FO. The rising incidence of breast cancer in women and prostate cancer in men. Dietary influences: a possible preventive role for nature's sex hormone modifiers-the phytoestrogens. *Oncol Rep* 1999 Jul-Aug;6(4):865-70

129.   Xu X, Duncan A. Effects of soy isoflavins an estrogen and phytoestrogen metabolism in premenopausal women. *Cancer Epidemiology Biomarkers Prev* 1998 Dec; 7(12):1101-8

130.   Goodman M, Wilkins L. Association of soy and fiber consumption with the risk of endometrial cancer. *Amer J of Epidemiology.* 1997 Aug 15; 146(4):294-306

131.   Potter S, Baum J. Soy protein and isoflavones: their effects on blood lipids and bone density in postmenopausal women. *Nutrition* 1998 Dec;68(6 Suppl):1375S-1379S

132.   Anderson JW, Johnstone BM. Meta-analysis of the effects of soy protein intake on serum lipids. *N Engl J Med* 1995 Aug 3;333(5):276-82

133.   Albertazzi P, Pansini F. Dietary soy supplementation and phytoestrogen levels. *Obstet Gynecol* 1999;94:229-31

HRT and Coronary Artery Disease

134.   Moerman CJ, Witteman JC. Hormone replacement therapy: a useful tool in the prevention of coronary artery disease in postmenopausal women? *Eur Menopause J.*1996; 3(2):60-68

135.   Ince C. Randomized trial of estrogen plus progestin for secondary prevention of coronary heart disease in postmenopausal women. *Medscape Cardiology*, 1998 (Abstract)

136.   Bush T. Effects of progestins on estrogen's cardioprotective benefits. Contemporary Ob/Gyn. 1998 Sep (Suppl): 18-26

137.   The writing group for the PEPI Trial. Effects of estrogen or estrogen/progestin regimens on heart disease risk factors in postmenopausal women. *JAMA.* 1995 an 18;273(3):199-208

138.   Heart and Estrogen/Progestin Replacement Study. *JAMA.* 1998;280:605-613

139.   Mercuro, G, Pitzalis L. Effects of acute administration of natural progesterone on peripheral vascular responsiveness in healthy postmenopausal women. *Am J Cardiol.* 1999 Jul 15; 84(2):214-218

140.   Miyagawa K, Rosch J. Medroxyprogesterone interferes with ovarian steroid protection against coronary vasospasm. Nature Medicine. 1997 Mar; 3 (3); 324-327

141. Matthews K, Kuller L. Prior use of estrogen replacement therapy, are users healthier than nonusers? *Am J Epidemiol.*1996; 143:971-8

142. Wenger N. HRT and coronary heart disease. *Womens Health in Primary Care.*1999;2(4):305-316

143. Notelovitz M. Adjustive estrogen therapy:a rational approach to HRT. *Contemporary Ob/Gyn.*1999 Feb:52-6

Resources

Salivary Hormone Testing

Diagnos-Techs, Inc.
Clinical & Research Laboratory
6620 S. 192nd Place, Bldg. J
Kent, Washington 98032
(800)-878-3787

Great Smokies Diagnostic Lab
63 Zillicoa St.
Asheville, NC 28801
(800) 522-4762 (for doctors) or (888) 891-3061 (for consumers)

Aeron Life Cycles
1933 Davis St. Suite 310
San Leandro, CA 94577
(800) 631-7900

ZRT Laboratory
12505 NW Cornell Rd.
Portland, OR 97213
(503) 469-0741

Soy Supplementation

Revival
Physicians Laboratories
Mail Order Only
(800) 500-2055
Ask a Physician
(800) 500-2055
www.revivalsoy.com
e-mail to doctors@revivalsoy.com

Organic Food Supplementation

Organic By Nature
P.O. Box 52561
Long Beach, CA 90832
(800) 362-8482
www.organicbynaturetrading.com

Natural Cosmetics, Progesterone Cream, Topical Pain Relief Creams

MW Labs
2002 Mills B. Lane Blvd
Savannah, GA 31405
(912) 236-9430
(912) 236-9338 Fax
www.mwlabs.com

Herbs and Vitamins

Metagenics
9503 E 55th Place
Tulsa, Oklahoma 74145
1-800 869-8100

PhytoPharmica Natural Medicines
(800) 553-2370
www.PhytoPharmica.com

Physicians Laboratories
Mail Order Only
(800) 500-2055
Ask a Physician
(800) 500-2055
www.revivalsoy.com
e-mail to doctors@revivalsoy.com

Compounding Pharmacy (Local)
To find a local compounding pharmacy contact:

Professional Compounding Centers of America (PCCA)

Phone: 800-331-2498 or 281-933-6948
Fax:　　800-874-5760 or 281-933-6627
Website: www.pccarx.com

Compounding Pharmacy(Mail Order)

Women's International Pharmacy
5708 Monona Drive
Madison, WI 53716-5708
(608)-221-7800; toll free (800) 279-5708

Are Your Hormones Making You Sick?

Contact the authors at
The Women's Wellness Group
5900 Hillandale Drive #325
Lithonia, Ga. 30058
(770) 981-4666
Website
www.areyourhormonesmakingyousick.com

e-mail:ebtmd@prodigy.net
or
www.wwgonline.net

The book is also available through Amazon.com,
BarnesNoble.com and all major bookstores.

Bulk orders can be purchased from
Biblio Distribution
Phone: 800-462-6420
Fax: 800-338-4550
www.bibliodistribution.com
E-Mail custserv@nbnbooks.com